HOME DOCTOR

KW-222-710

AN A-Z GUIDE

HOME DOCTOR

AN A-Z GUIDE

by Dr Victor G. Daniels

BSc, PhD, MB, BChir, Dip.Pharm.Med.

Cambridge Medical Books
Cambridge, England

Published by
Cambridge Medical Books
Tracey Hall
Cockburn Street
Cambridge CB1 3NB
England
Tel 0223 212423

ISBN 0 948920 02 5

Copyright © 1986 Victor G. Daniels

All rights reserved. No part of this publication may be
reproduced, stored in retrieval system, or transmitted in any
form or by any means, electronic, mechanical, photocopying,
recording or otherwise, without prior permission from the
publisher.

Typeset and printed by Heffers Printers Ltd, Cambridge,
England

Preface

This book is a non-technical reference source, bringing together clearly and concisely information about common ailments and their treatment. An easy-to-read A–Z format allows it to be kept handy for quick and easy reference at all times. It provides useful advice on how to cope with everyday illnesses. Each ailment or condition is considered under the following headings: Definition, Home Treatment and Seek Medical Advice.

Advice is therefore offered on how much can be done in the home and more importantly when to seek medical advice. An appendix provides information on self-help organisations, classification of drugs, surgical operations and normal heights and weights of children and adults.

Before publication the manuscript was extensively reviewed by several pharmacists and general practitioners. I am grateful to the following for their helpful comments and suggestions. Christine Chard, Kathy Piper, Vernon Thompson and Dr. Sidney Hopkins kindly commented from the pharmacy viewpoint. Dr. Tim Moriarty and Dr. Ian Parker commented from the general practitioner viewpoint. Finally I am indebted to my wife Ruth for her excellent proof reading, to the staff at Family Circle for encouragement and support and to Gill Norman who skillfully word processed the manuscript.

No book is without flaw and I would be very pleased to receive suggestions which readers think might help to make future editions more valuable.

DR VICTOR G. DANIELS

Cambridge
April 1986

Emergency Information

Doctor
Surgery Address

Telephone No.

Surgery Hours

Night Service

Alternative Doctor
Telephone No.

Hospitals
Address

Telephone No's.

Pharmacists
Telephone No's.

Medical Insurance Company
Address

Telephone No.
Policy No.

Ambulance

Fire

Police

Taxi Services
Telephone No's.

Dentist
Address

Telephone No

Other Specialists and Consultants

Person to contact in emergency
Address

Telephone No.

Miscellaneous

CONTENTS

DEFINITION

- Acne is a very common skin condition usually of the face, neck, upper chest and back that affects teenagers and young adults.
- It is caused by blockage and infection of the sebaceous or oil glands in the skin.
- In mild cases there may be only blackheads and small pimples; in severe cases these spots may be filled with pus or even turn into cysts.
- Acne is not infectious.

HOME TREATMENT

- Cleanliness – wash the areas affected twice daily with a medicated soap and hot water – this helps to keep the skin pores open and remove layers of oil (sebum).
- Avoid greases and waxes on the skin.
- Never squeeze or try to remove spots – it can leave disfiguring scars.
- Shave with an electric razor rather than a blade.
- A holiday in the sun or an ultraviolet lamp is helpful.
- Keep hair away from the forehead thus allowing sunlight to the skin.
- There are no dietary restrictions – chocolates, nuts, sweets and spicey food do not make acne worse.
- Your pharmacist will advise you on medicated soaps as well as on the availability of a number of proprietary lotions and creams. These produce a mild peeling effect and so lift material out of the skin pores.

. . . *continued*

SEEK MEDICAL ADVICE

- Your doctor may prescribe a course of antibiotics which you may need to take regularly for a prolonged period – around six months or so.
- You may be referred for a specialist opinion to a dermatologist (skin doctor).
- Some oral contraceptive pills may aggravate acne, others improve acne – ask your doctor.
- Usually acne clears itself in adult life – sooner or later it will improve – but do not expect an immediate response to treatment.

ALLERGY

DEFINITION

- An unusual sensitivity by a part of the body to some substances (eg foodstuffs, pollen, dust, jewellery, cosmetics, insects, medicines, animal fur) which are normally well tolerated by other people.
- Common examples of allergic reactions include asthma, hay fever, allergic rhinitis (runny nose), nettle rash and eczema (see also Eczema).
- Symptoms include itchy, red skin, red and itchy eyes, runny nose, difficulty breathing (asthma) due to the narrowing of airways.

HOME TREATMENT

- Avoid causative agents, eg foodstuffs or pollen.

SEEK MEDICAL ADVICE

- Skin tests may help to discover allergic substances and it may be possible to have a desensitising course of injections. Your doctor may prescribe medicines, eg antihistamines or, more rarely, steroids for general allergic conditions.
- For asthma your doctor may prescribe inhalers or tablets.

ANAL PAIN, ITCHING AND BLEEDING

DEFINITION
- Piles (haemorrhoids) are small swollen blood vessels and may appear as a lump at the anus.
- They may cause irritation, pain or bleeding.
- There are broadly two types of piles: those arising internally inside the rectum and those arising externally outside the anus. Both types may occur together.

HOME TREATMENT
- Many cases of piles respond to home treatment.
- Keep the area clean – use a shower or bidet regularly and dry carefully afterwards. Hygienic wipes or pads may be useful.
- Hot baths or hot compresses can help to relieve the pain.
- Avoid scratching.
- Keep bowel motions soft – avoid constipation. Eat plenty of vegetables and bran. If not effective ask your pharmacist for his advice on laxatives.
- Dry the area carefully then apply a barrier cream such as zinc and castor oil around the anus.
- Internal haemorrhoids may be helped by a suppository – ask your pharmacist for advice.
- Piles may occur in pregnancy but usually disappear after birth.

SEEK MEDICAL ADVICE
- If bleeding, pain or a rash does not resolve after a week with home treatment.
- Your doctor may refer you to a surgeon for further treatment.

ANKLES – SWOLLEN

DEFINITION
- Ankle swelling is a common problem that may occur in people who are on their feet a lot during the day.
- Mild ankle swelling is also a fairly common feature during pregnancy.

HOME TREATMENT
- Avoid tight clothing – especially garters.
- Avoid prolonged standing or sitting.
- If this is not possible then, while standing or sitting, exercise leg muscles by curling toes, tightening–up calf muscles and massage.
- When possible, sit or lie with legs elevated.
- If possible lose weight.
- Avoid smoking.

SEEK MEDICAL ADVICE
- If ankle swelling is sudden and is accompanied by breathlessness or by pain and redness of the skin.
- If caused by an injury (see Sprains).

ANXIETY AND STRESS

DEFINITION

- Anxiety is an expression of 'tension' or 'stress' that may range in intensity from mild to panic.
- It is the most common of all emotional reactions.
- In a small minority of cases anxiety may be a symptom of disease.

HOME TREATMENT

- Understand your own feelings of tension and anxiety, these can be manifested for example by increased sweating, nausea, vomiting and diarrhoea, frequent passing of urine, headache, dizzy spells and insomnia, interference with work or social relationships.
- Discover how best to cope with life's problems;for example decrease the amount of unfinished business your mind is 'carrying'.
- If the cause of your anxiety cannot be removed, learn to cope with it and accept things as they are, at least for now.
- Talk about your problems with friends and relatives – they might be able to provide reassurance.
- Try relaxation techniques like meditation, yoga, exercise, hypnosis etc.
- Take up a hobby like walking or fishing and set aside enough time to enjoy it.

SEEK MEDICAL ADVICE

- If your symptoms worry you excessively. The doctor will reassure you if there is no physical cause for your anxiety.
- He may prescribe a short course of a mild tranquilliser or sedative to help you cope better with the stress and so break the vicious cycle of worry.

ATHLETE'S FOOT

DEFINITION
- Athletes foot is a fungal infection of the skin which thrives in warm, damp conditions.
- It is commonly found between the toes and on the soles of the feet and may produce itching, flaking, blistering and cracking of the skin.

HOME TREATMENT
- Foot hygiene – keep feet clean and dry, especially between the toes. Wash the space between the toes twice a day with soap and water. Dry carefully with a towel and change socks frequently.
- Avoid tight fitting footwear and wear open sandals whenever possible or, better still, go barefoot.
- Your pharmacist will recommend an antifungal cream, powder or ointment for use until the skin between the toes is clear of the infection.
- Apply both cream and powder. Use the cream at least twice a day and dust the shoes and socks with powder.
- Treatment should be continued for one week after the symptoms have disappeared. This is to try and prevent reinfection which is common.

SEEK MEDICAL ADVICE
- If self–treatment has not helped or if the diagnosis is uncertain.
- Your doctor may prescribe other cream or ointment or an antifungal drug to be taken by mouth particularly if you have a persistent infection.

BACK PAIN

DEFINITION

- Back pain is a common complaint and is the major cause of lost work time in Britain. It usually involves spasm or strain of the big supportive muscles that run alongside the spine. The great majority of cases recover within one to four weeks.

HOME TREATMENT

- ACUTE BACK PAIN
- Lie flat on firm, level surface.
- Take a pain relieving drug for example paracetamol, ibuprofen or aspirin every 4 hours until the symptoms subside.
- Be patient – it may be several hours before it improves and up to a few weeks before you are back to normal.
- Heat supplied to the area can provide some relief – use a covered hot water bottle or an infra–red lamp for short periods. Portable thermal packs are available – ask your pharmacist.
- CHRONIC BACK PAIN
- Improve posture, aiming to keep the lower back straight or curved slightly backwards for most of the time.
- Keep fit and supple – swimming and yoga may help, as may simple back exercises.
- Don't get overweight.
- Avoid heavy lifting but when you do lift, bend your knees and keep your back straight and, if moving with a load, move your feet rather than swivel your hips or shoulders.
- Wear low heeled shoes.
- Avoid unnecessary standing but when you have to stand or sit at a table or desk, try to rest one foot at least 6 inches off the ground on an empty box.

. . . continued

- Put a hard–board under your mattress or buy an orthopaedic bed.
- Take a pain relieving drug for example paracetamol, ibuprofen or aspirin up to four times a day until the symptoms subside.

SEEK MEDICAL ADVICE

- If the pain results from a recent injury or the pain travels down one or both legs below the knee.
- If back pain is associated with any change in sensation or weakness in the legs.
- Your doctor may refer you to a physiotherapist for further treatment.
- Many doctors recognise that osteopaths and chiropractors also play a useful role in the treatment of back pain, and your doctor may be willing to refer you.

BAD BREATH (HALITOSIS)

DEFINITION

- Bad breath may be caused by a number of conditions; sore throat, catarrh, sinusitis, chest infections and, more commonly, dental and gum disorders.

HOME TREATMENT

- Check with your partner or friend that there is a problem.
- Stop smoking – take plenty of exercise in the open air.
- Cut down drink especially alcohol and coffee.
- Avoid spiced foods that include, onions, garlic etc.
- Take extra care with teeth and gums, as well as brushing teeth regularly, use dental floss or a tooth pick to remove debris between teeth. If necessary consult a dentist.
- Use a mild antiseptic mouthwash or gel.

SEEK MEDICAL ADVICE

- If halitosis still remains after any obvious cause is removed.

BEDWETTING (ENURESIS)

DEFINITION

- The age at which a child becomes 'dry' at night is usually during the second and third years.
- Bedwetting is a common occurrence and about 10% of 5 – 6 year olds wet their beds.
- In the great majority of cases no significant abnormality is found.

HOME TREATMENT

- Only toilet–train a child when he shows signs of being ready.
- Never use punishment to aid toilet training.
- Try not to be over anxious about the problem since it may well make your child worse.
- Give praise for dry nights.
- Offer small prizes or treats for dry beds – use a star chart to show which have been dry nights.
- Make sure your child goes to the toilet just before bedtime.
- Avoid late night drinking and eating.
- Occasionally special pads with alarms may be used – the bell rings when the pad becomes wet and wakes the child in time to get up and use the toilet.

SEEK MEDICAL ADVICE

- If a child after the age of 4 years is wet by day and night.
- Your doctor may request a specimen of urine to check for infection.
- Usually no cause is found but your doctor may decide to prescribe a short course of a drug to help lessen wetting.

BITES AND STINGS

DEFINITION

- Bites and stings by animals or insects are unfortunately an unavoidable hazard of everyday life.

HOME TREATMENT

- Remove sting if visible by forcing it out with thumb nail or tweezers. Never pull it out.
- Scrub wound clean with soap and water and clean out regularly with soap and water or a mild antiseptic 2–3 times a day for 2–3 days.
- For an insect bite or sting apply something cold – ice or cold packs may be used.
- Bees and ants have acid venom so apply the alkali, sodium bicarbonate (baking powder)to the sting.
- Wasps and hornets have alkali venom so apply acidic lemon or vinegar.
- If painful, take aspirin or paracetamol every 4 hours until symptoms subside.
- Your pharmacist will advise you about antihistamine creams and tablets that may help to reduce the swelling and itching.
- If a limb is swollen, elevate the limb to help drain excess tissue fluid away from the area that's been affected.
- Avoid scratching, since dirt introduced into a bite or sting may produce an infection.
- Relieve local irritation by applying calamine lotion.

. . . continued

SEEK MEDICAL ADVICE

- **IMMEDIATELY** if there are symptoms of an allergic reaction – shock, collapse, difficulty with breathing.
- If wound is deep since it may require stitching. A tetanus injection may also be required.
- Tetanus booster injection is needed every 5 years to prevent tetanus.
- If you are bitten by an animal when travelling abroad, seek medical advice on the need for rabies inoculation after first receiving first aid.

BLEEDING GUMS

DEFINITION

- Bleeding from the gums when the teeth are brushed usually clears up in a short while if attention is paid to proper teeth cleaning.
- A common cause of bleeding gums is bacterial plaque. Early inflammation is called gingivitis.

HOME TREATMENT

- Check toothbrush – it may be too hard.
- Too vigorous or too frequent brushing can make the gums bleed. Use a small-headed medium soft toothbrush.
- Eat plenty of fresh fruit if fruit is not a regular part of your diet.
- Use an antiseptic mouthwash or gel.
- If profuse bleeding occurs after a tooth extraction make a pad from a piece of gauze or a handkerchief and bite hard on it for 10–15 minutes.

SEEK MEDICAL ADVICE

- If the condition does not clear up with home treatment since the gums may be infected.
- If you notice bruising or bleeding elsewhere on your body.

DEFINITION

- A boil (abscess) is an infection of the skin in which pus forms. It is usually caused by bacteria and often starts around a hair root.
- A carbuncle is a collection of boils.

HOME TREATMENT

- Apply hot soaks; these may help a boil to come to a head quicker.
- Do not squeeze the boil – handle it gently – since the infection can be forced deeper into the skin.
- Your pharmacist can provide you with magnesium sulphate paste which is applied to the area and covered with a dressing. This acts as a poultice and draws the infection towards the surface to a 'head'.
- Once the boil has ruptured apply warm moist soaks to ensure full drainage of the pus.
- Use own towels and face flannels and keep separately.

SEEK MEDICAL ADVICE

- If the boil is large or painful and home treatment has failed.
- If boils are recurrent, as antibiotics may be needed and urine should be tested for sugar to exclude the possibility of diabetes.
- Your doctor may decide to lance or cut into the boil to ensure proper drainage.

BREAST LUMPS

DEFINITION

- Most lumps in the breast are harmless areas of fatty tissue or cysts but nevertheless a lump should be examined by a doctor as soon as it is detected.

HOME TREATMENT

- Examine the breasts regularly at the same time each month. For example after each period.
- If your periods have stopped, examine the breasts about once a month.
- To examine the breasts:
  a. Undress to the waist and stand in front of a mirror. Look at the breasts with arms down by your sides and then with arms raised. The breasts are often different in size and you should note any change since the last examination.
  b. Lie on the back and feel each breast starting at the armpit with the flat of the opposite hand. Do this once with the arm down by the side and then with the arm raised above the head. Feel each part of each breast in turn, moving round in a circle.
  c. Make sure to look under each breast for puckering or any other unusual changes.

SEEK MEDICAL ADVICE

- If you find a lump or swelling which is still present after the period.
- If there is skin trouble around the nipple or 'pulling in' of the nipple so that it becomes inverted.
- If there is a stained discharge from the nipple.
- If there is pain in the breast not confined to the time just before a period.
- Your GP may refer you to a specialist for some investigations.

BRUISES

DEFINITION

- Bruising is caused by the release of blood from damaged blood vessels into the tissues, following injury.
- The discolouration is initially blue, purple or black but fades to yellow as the blood is broken down and removed from the skin.

HOME TREATMENT

- General Advice:
  I – Immobilisation
  C – Compression
  E – Elevation
- If painful take a painkiller for example paracetamol or aspirin until symptoms subside.
- Apply ice packs or cold compresses, lint wrung out in ice–cold water.
- Witch hazel lotion may provide some relief.

SEEK MEDICAL ADVICE

- If bruising persists or is extensive.
- If bruising occurs without an external injury.

BUNIONS

DEFINITION

- A bunion is a harmless inflammation of the small sac of fluid (bursa) at the base of the big toes caused by wearing too tight shoes.
- Bunions are more common in women than men, and usually affect both feet.

HOME TREATMENT

- Ensure shoes fit properly.
- Avoid high heels.
- Avoid wearing shoes with pointed toes.
- Take care choosing shoes and avoid direct pressure on the joint. Use adhesive cushion pads or moleskin inside footwear (available from the pharmacist).
- Foot exercises such as picking up marbles with the toes may help.
- A chiropodist may help to relieve discomfort.
- Bunions are usually painful and painkillers may need to be taken regularly eg aspirin or paracetamol.

SEEK MEDICAL ADVICE

- If the bunion is very painful or if it becomes red and inflamed or discharges.

BURNS AND SCALDS

DEFINITION

- In mild burns or first–degree burns there may be only reddening of the skin. In second–degree burns there is blistering and splitting of the skin layers. Third–degree burns destroy all layers of the skin and extend into the deeper tissues.

HOME TREATMENT

FIRST/SECOND DEGREE ONLY:
- Flood burnt area with cold running water or immerse in cold water for at least 10 minutes.
- Do not attempt to remove burnt clothing from the damaged area.
- Do not prick or rupture blisters.

THIRD DEGREE ONLY:
- Cover burnt area with non–adherent dressing or dry clean cloth.
- Do not apply water.
- Seek urgent medical advice.

GENERAL:
- Superficial burns like sunburn do not require dressing; they usually heal well.
- Take a painkiller for example paracetamol or aspirin until symptoms subside.
- If area is weeping, keep as clean as possible to avoid any risk of infection.

SEEK MEDICAL ADVICE

- IMMEDIATELY if patient is shocked or collapses – lie the casualty on the floor, keep warm and treat for shock. (See Shock)
- If the burn is deep or if any burn is still painful after 24 hours of self–treatment.

CATARRH

DEFINITION
- A vague term that implies a "stuffed–up" feeling in the head and nose.
- Catarrhal episodes are usually harmless and self–limiting.

HOME TREATMENT
- Don't smoke.
- Regular nose–blowing may be of some help.
- Use inhalations such as friar's balsam or menthol crystals. Simply add boiling water to the preparation and put a towel over your head and inhale the vapour for 5 minutes.
- Nasal drops and sprays, like inhalations also help to break up or liquefy the secretions. Ask your pharmacist for advice.
- Do not use nasal drops or sprays for too long or too often as they can make the symptoms worse.
- Preparations are also available to reduce the production of mucus.

SEEK MEDICAL ADVICE
- If catarrh persists and causes unpleasant problems such as nasal blockage or breathlessness.
- If catarrh occurs in summer only or on exposure to dusts – it's possible an allergy could be present.

CHICKENPOX

DEFINITION
- Chickenpox is a common viral infective illness of childhood, a second attack is rare.
- The same virus also causes shingles (see Shingles) and in an individual who has had chickenpox the virus may lie dormant in the body for years and shingles may develop later in life.
- The typical rash goes from red blotches and bumps to small blisters which later form a crust.

HOME TREATMENT
- Incubation period is usually 10–21 days. By the time the crusts appear the disease is no longer infectious.
- Keep children away from school for one week after the rash first appears.
- Apply calamine lotion twice daily to soothe the itching.
- Proprietary preparations are available that act to 'seal' the spots. Ask your pharmacist for advice.
- Lukewarm baths are usually helpful.
- Avoid scratching as this may lead to infection of the blisters and may produce permanent scars.
- Painkillers such as aspirin or paracetamol may be required in severe cases.
- If sleep is disturbed by intense itching you can give an antihistamine e.g. Phenergan syrup.
- When spots are inside the mouth gargling with salt water (half a teaspoon to a glass of warm water) helps.
- Elderly people should avoid close contact since they may develop shingles.

SEEK MEDICAL ADVICE
- If not sure of diagnosis or if child appears to be ill.
- If not clearing up after 7–10 days.

CHILBLAINS

DEFINITION

- A red painful and itching area usually affecting the feet, hands and nose, after exposure to the cold.
- Some people seem to be particularly susceptible.

HOME TREATMENT

- Avoid sudden changes of skin temperature during the winter.
- In cold weather wear good protective clothing over the hands and feet.
- Wear comfortable but not too tight footwear and gloves.
- Keep skin clean and dry and try to avoid injuries which break the skin.
- Do not rub the chilblain or warm suddenly – but warm the area gradually.
- Do not scratch the chilblains.
- Creams and tablets are available from your pharmacist to help prevent and treat chilblains.

SEEK MEDICAL ADVICE

- If chilblains are persistent or severe or if a skin infection develops, if you are elderly, diabetic or suffer from arthritis of the hands or feet.
- Your doctor may prescribe a medicine that helps with the circulation particularly to the hands and feet.

CHILD ABUSE

There are over 8000 cases of non–accidental injury reported in England each year and these result in over 100 deaths.

SYMPTOMS
- Child may be thin, under–nourished and unhappy with many unexplained absences from school.
- Bruising: on body, and face – black eye.
- Pinch and grip marks.
- Bite marks.
- Strap or imprint marks.
- Burns: scalds, cigarette burns.
- Mouth injuries: teeth, torn ligament of tongue.
- Bone injuries (skull, humerous, rib etc).
- Internal injuries: ruptured liver or spleen etc.

WHAT TO DO
- Local education authority usually issue detailed instruction.
- Through LEA inform general practitioner of your suspicions.
- Contact social services through the Education Welfare Officer.
- If parents are uncooperative the doctor can arrange for Place of Safety Order (via Social Services Department and NSPCC – see below).

TWO MAJOR ACTS PROVIDE FOR THE CARE OF YOUNG PERSONS
- Child Care Act 1980. Covers children whose parents are temporarily or permanently, unable to care for them adequately and who place their children voluntarily into the keeping of the local authority.

. . . continued

- Children and Young Persons Act 1969. Under the 1969 Act a local authority can apply to a juvenile court for an order allowing it to remove a child from its parents' care where the child's health or development is being 'avoidably impaired or neglected' or the child is being ill–treated.

USEFUL ADDRESSES

- National Advisory Centre on the Battered Child
  Denver House
  The Drive
  Bounds Green Road
  LONDON N1
  Tel: 01 361 1181

COLDS AND FLU

DEFINITION

- A frequent self–limiting illness caused by a number of different highly contagious viruses.
- The virus affects the upper respiratory tract producing a swollen and inflamed lining of the nose, sinuses, and throat.
- The illness usually lasts for up to seven days with or without treatment.

HOME TREATMENT

- Where possible carry on with normal activities unless you are feeling ill or feverish.
- Take plenty of hot drinks to replace the fluid lost by extra sweating.
- Do not smoke and avoid tobacco fumes.
- Take painkillers e.g. aspirin or paracetamol regularly until symptoms subside. Cold remedies also help to ease nasal symptoms. Some of these preparations may also help you sleep. Ask your pharmacist for his advice.
- If you have dry cough take plenty of hot drinks or simple cough medicines such as codeine linctus.
- Extra sleep or bed–rest helps recovery.
- The cold virus does not respond to antibiotics nor to any other drugs so do not request these from your doctor. Your body will eventually destroy the virus.

SEEK MEDICAL ADVICE

- If the symptoms do not clear within a few days or if the cold has gone onto the chest or into the ears or sinuses.

COLD EXTREMITIES (RAYNAUD'S DISEASE)

DEFINITION

- Raynaud's disease is a condition where small blood vessels carrying blood to the 'extremities' (usually the fingers) have constricted. As a result the fingers become white and numb.
- It is quite a common condition especially among women.

HOME TREATMENT

- Keep warm at all times with loose socks and gloves, particularly before going outside.
- Wear comfortable roomy footwear. Try to keep hands in a low position (below level of heart).
- Take care of infections around the nails since they may take quite a long time to heal.
- Avoid smoking.
- Avoid excessive use of hand held power tools, as vibration can cause narrowing of blood vessels.

SEEK MEDICAL ADVICE

- If problem persists despite keeping warm or if there are any other important symptoms.
- The doctor may prescribe a drug that helps the circulation or he may refer you for a specialist opinion which could involve surgery of the nerves that cause blood vessels to contract (called a sympathectomy).

COLD SORES

DEFINITION

- Cold sores found on the lips and around the mouth are usually caused by a virus called herpes simplex.
- The virus lies dormant in the nerves under the skin and flares up possibly with a cold, over–exposure to sunlight, sea air or cold weather, periods, or for no obvious reason.
- The same group of viruses causes genital herpes.
- The cold sore may start with prickling or itching in the area with the sores appearing within 10 days.

HOME TREATMENT

- Apply a little surgical spirit or camphor spirit on cotton wool every 3 or 4 hours until cleared, or use a special proprietary product available from your pharmacist.
- Rinse out your mouth frequently with an antiseptic mouthwash.
- Do not squeeze the sores – the infection may spread by the fingers to other parts of the face.
- Wash hands well – use your own towels and keep them separate.
- Healing normally occurs within 7–10 days but recurrence is unfortunately always possible.

SEEK MEDICAL ADVICE

- If the cold sores are recurrent or severe, or if the rash is near the eye.
- Your doctor may prescribe an anti–viral liquid or cream to paint onto the sores.

COLIC

DEFINITION

- Describes the intermittent spasms of pain originating from the intestines. It happens more commonly in young babies and generally stops after the age of three months.
- It may occur periodically in adults.

HOME TREATMENT FOR ADULTS

- If pain is troublesome avoid food. Take sips of water only.
- Sit or lie down in a comfortable position.
- A hot water bottle applied to the painful area may help.

- Proprietary liquids and tablets are available from your pharmacist.

SEEK MEDICAL ADVICE

- If pain is severe and recurrent and if associated with a generalised illness e.g. fever or diarrhoea.

CONJUNCTIVITIS

DEFINITION

- Conjunctivitis is an inflammation or infection of the conjunctival membrane that lines the white of the eye and the inner surface of the eyelids. It is sometimes contagious and it is easily spread to the other eye.
- It may be caused by an irritant e.g. chlorine in swimming pool water, an allergy to something in the air e.g. pollen, or by bacteria or a virus.

HOME TREATMENT

- Rest the eyes while avoiding bright lights; do not cover the eye with an eye patch.
- Bathe the eye in warm saline water (one level teaspoon of salt to a pint of boiled water) or an eye lotion.
- Your pharmacist may recommend an eye lotion.
- Avoid any known irritants, e.g. chlorine in water, tobacco smoke, pollen etc.
- The patient should use his own towel and flannel as bacterial and viral conjunctivitis can spread rapidly.

SEEK MEDICAL ADVICE

- If there is severe pain in the eye rather than itching, burning or grittiness or if there is any difficulty with vision.
- If there is a thick discharge or if the eye symptoms do not settle within 48 hours.
- The doctor may prescribe antibiotic ointment or drops to be put into the eyes frequently.

CONSTIPATION

DEFINITION

- Irregular or difficult bowel movements.
- Many people are preoccupied with their bowels! Bowel movements may occur three times a day or once every three days, both are normal.

HOME TREATMENT

- Eat a balanced diet with plenty of roughage, including fresh fruit, vegetables, nuts, cereals, natural unprocessed bran.
- Bran may be used in baking or mixed with other food, or it can be used to thicken sauces or soups etc.
- Drink plenty of fluids, especially natural fruit juices.
- Take regular exercise and plenty of fresh air.
- Develop a healthy disregard for details of bowel actions.
- Proprietary laxatives, purgatives or suppositories may be helpful if constipation is causing pain but avoid regular use – no more than for a few days at a time. Ask your pharmacist for advice.

SEEK MEDICAL ADVICE

- If there is a major change in bowel habit or if there is blood in the stools.

COUGH

DEFINITION

- The cough reflex is a normal protective or defence mechanism that eliminates excess secretions and inhaled foreign bodies such as dust from the chest.
- A cough does not always require treatment.

HOME TREATMENT

- Don't smoke and keep away from smoke.
- Take a cough medicine containing one or a mixture of a antihistamine or cough suppressant or expectorants may be helpful. The pharmacist will advise you.
- Try hot, sweet drinks or simple cough linctuses.
- Steam inhalations mixed with menthol, eucalyptus or friar's balsam may help – ask the pharmacist.
- If the cough is dry and distressing it may require treatment.

SEEK MEDICAL ADVICE

- If coughing is accompanied by high fever, pains in the chest, wheezing, breathlessness or blood stained phlegm.
- If cough persists for more than 1–2 weeks.
- If coughing up a yellow–green – coloured phlegm. An antibiotic will probably be prescribed.

CRADLE CAP (BABY DANDRUFF)

DEFINITION

- Cradle cap is common in young infants and consists of small areas of yellowish brown discolouration and crusting on the scalp that resembles dandruff.
- The cause is excess scalp grease, together with insufficient washing and brushing.

HOME TREATMENT

- Apply a mild medicated shampoo which loosens scales regularly. Ask your pharmacist for advice.
- Brush and comb the affected areas with a soft brush.

SEEK MEDICAL ADVICE

- If severe and not improving with home treatment.
- Your doctor can prescribe special shampoos and lotions if necessary.

CRAMP

DEFINITION

- Cramp is a condition caused by painful muscle spasm usually of the leg. It may be caused by overexertion, poor muscular coordination or excessive sweating in very hot weather.
- It does not cause permanent damage though muscles may be tender and stiff for a few days.

HOME TREATMENT

- Warm, rub and gently stretch the cramped muscle. Application of embrocations or lotion may help.
- Try to straighten the affected muscle immediately the cramp begins.
- Take calcium tablets or, especially for cramp in hot climates, salt tablets – ask your pharmacist.
- For night cramps in the elderly, tablets may help – ask your pharmacist.
- If subject to cramps do not swim out of your depth.

SEEK MEDICAL ADVICE

- If sleep is being seriously impaired or if troublesome attacks continue.

CROUP

DEFINITION
- Croup is an infectious viral condition that results in partial obstruction of the voice box (larynx) that occurs mainly in children and is characterised by a barking cough and difficulty in breathing.

HOME TREATMENT
- A warm, steamy atmosphere, e.g. kitchen or bathroom with kettle boiling or hot tap running relieves the symptoms.
- Give the child a warm drink and then reassure and comfort.
- Make sure that the bedroom is warm and the air made moist by leaving a bowl of water in the room before taking the child back into the room. Commercial vapourisers are also available. Ask the pharmacist.
- You can usually cope with mild attacks by the use of steam inhalations which should be handled very carefully.

SEEK MEDICAL ADVICE
- IMMEDIATELY if the attack is severe and the child is very breathless.
- The doctor may prescribe an antibiotic or if concerned he may admit the child to hospital for further treatment and observation.

CUTS AND GRAZES

DEFINITION

- Minor cuts and grazes do not require any treatment unless infection has set in the wound.

HOME TREATMENT

- Stop bleeding – apply firm pressure on bleeding area.
- Gently clean the wound thoroughly with soap and water – use a clean soft nail brush, if necessary, to get all the dirt out.
- Wipe outwards and away from the cut.
- A cleansing agent e.g. hydrogen peroxide helps to lift the dirt out.
- Apply an antiseptic cream or ointment.
- Apply a dry dressing.
- If wound is wide, use sticking plaster to draw the edges of the wound together.

SEEK MEDICAL ADVICE

- If bleeding cannot be controlled.
- If a wound is deep, becomes infected or if you cannot get all the dirt out of it.
- A tetanus injection may be required. Tetanus booster injections are needed every 5 years.

CYSTITIS

DEFINITION

- Cystitis is a condition where there is burning and frequent passing of urine.
- Cystitis is an infection or inflammation of the lining of the bladder and is common in newly married women (honeymoon cystitis) and pregnant women.
- Most women will experience an attack of cystitis sometime in their life.
- An attack of cystitis in men and children is uncommon and should be referred to a doctor.

HOME TREATMENT

- Drink a lot of fluids (half a pint every 20 minutes for at least 3 hours daily) to help flush away the infection from the bladder.
- Empty the bladder frequently.
- Avoid alcohol and coffee which can irritate the bladder lining.
- Take one teaspoonful of bicarbonate of soda in a glass of water 3 times a day for 2–3 days or until the symptoms subside. Bicarbonate of soda and potassium citrate make the urine less acid and helps to stop bacteria multiplying.
- Potassium citrate sachets are also available from your pharmacist.
- If burning is severe take painkillers for example aspirin or paracetamol until symptoms subside.
- A hot water bottle wrapped in a towel applied over the area is comforting.
- For recurrent cystitis in women simple measures may help –
  a. Wash external genitals with non–medicated unperfumed soap and water twice daily.

. . . continued

b. Do not use vaginal deodorants or bubble baths, shampoos, bath oils etc.

c. Wipe toilet tissues from front to back so fewer bacteria are spread from the back passage.

d. Wear cotton pants and avoid tights and tight trousers.

e. In cold weather wear warm underclothing and trousers rather than skirts.

f. Empty bladder if possible about 10–15 minutes after sexual intercourse, and wash area.

SEEK MEDICAL ADVICE

- If symptoms persist for more than 24 – 48 hours an antibiotic may be needed or if blood is passed in the urine as further investigation may be required.
- If you are pregnant.

DANDRUFF

DEFINITION

- Dandruff is a common skin problem and refers to the fine white dry scales found on the scalp of people with the condition.
- Dandruff is often at its worst during adolescence but it may occur at other ages.

HOME TREATMENT

- Keep your hair clean – avoid waxes or greases.
- Use a medicated or detergent shampoo – ask your pharmacist for his advice.
- Follow the instructions carefully.
- Most cases respond to home treatment.

SEEK MEDICAL ADVICE

- If the condition does not respond to home treatment or if the scalp becomes infected.

DEPRESSION

DEFINITION
- Depression is a very unpleasant experience that may include some or all of the following symptoms:
  - Feelings of guilt
  - Apathy and poor work performance
  - Lack of energy as well as loss of appetite
  - Insomnia and early morning waking
  - Mood variations
  - Lack of interest in sex and life generally

HOME TREATMENT
- Not all types of depression need medical treatment – there is much that can be done to treat depression if its cause is obvious for example housing, social or marital problems etc.
- Seek help and reassurance from your friends and family.
- Try and carry on with a normal life.
- Your priest or minister or a qualified hypnotherapist, or self–help groups can provide support.
- Marriage guidance counselling is available to married and unmarried people. (See local telephone book for nearest branch)
- You can speak to the Samaritans on the telephone – they can be phoned at any time.
- Mild cases of depression usually get better in time without drug treatment.

SEEK MEDICAL ADVICE
- If depression is without any obvious cause.
- If you feel suicidal.
- Your doctor may prescribe a short course of an anti–depressant drug which will help you cope with day–to–day activities.
- You may be referred to a specialist for treatment.

DIARRHOEA

DEFINITION
- A fairly common disorder caused by a wide variety of conditions. The most usual causes are dietary indiscretion and emotional upset.
- Babies and the elderly are at special risk because of the dangers caused by fluid loss from excessive diarrhoea.

HOME TREATMENT
- Avoid all solid food for at least 24 hours. Drink water or soft drinks – a small amount regularly say every hour.
- Avoid milk, substitute boiled water or fruit juices for babies (it does not harm at all not to eat for two to three days so long as fluids are taken regularly).
- Gradually try to return to your normal diet over the next few days.
- Your pharmacist may give you a mixture of kaolin and morphine to treat the diarrhoea, or a proprietary preparation if rapid control is needed. Alternatively hc may provide you with a proprietary glucose–salt solution.

SEEK MEDICAL ADVICE
- If diarrhoea is severe and associated with pain and if it persists for more than three days.
- If the patient is a baby, a small child or an elderly person.
- If associated with generalised illness.
- If motion contains blood or slime.
- If the patient has recently returned from abroad.

DIZZINESS AND UNSTEADINESS

DEFINITION

- Vertigo or 'true dizziness' is caused by a disturbance in the balance mechanism of the inner ear.
- The patient feels he or the room is spinning round.
- Nausea and vomiting may also occur.

HOME TREATMENT

- Move slowly, do not suddenly change your posture, especially on getting out of bed or on lying down.
- In particular do not suddenly turn your head or look up – this may bring on attacks.
- Do not attempt to carry on with your job or driving.
- Try and relax since emotional upset can bring on an 'attack' of dizziness.
- Taking preparations for motion sickness may help – ask your pharmacist for advice.

SEEK MEDICAL ADVICE

- If the attacks are frequent or last for more than a day or so.
- If attacks are associated with ear problems or any loss of hearing.

EAR, NOISES IN (TINNITUS)

DEFINITION

- Tinnitus is a condition in which the sufferer is aware of a distressing noise such as ringing or buzzing in the ears or head that has no external cause.
- The noises are usually loudest when the environment is quiet.
- The most common type of noise is a single pure tone like a ring or a whistle. Noises like escaping steam or rushing water are also common.

HOME TREATMENT

- Wax may be the cause: use olive oil or almond oil drops to try and soften it or the pharmacist may recommend a proprietary preparation.
- Use other noises to mask out the distressing tinnitus. For example keep a radio on in the background all the time even when going to sleep.
- A tinnitus ear insert (maskers), available from a hearing aid specialist, may help. These maskers make 'white noise' which is comforting to sufferers.
- No pills or medicines will make any difference to the condition. High doses of some medicines for example aspirin or quinine actually cause tinnitus.

SEEK MEDICAL ADVICE

- If noises persist for more than a few days as there may be ear disease or hard wax present.
- When tinnitus is combined with giddiness and deafness this is known as Meniere's disease and requires medical attention.

EAR WAX

DEFINITION

- Wax in the outer canal of the ear is a very common problem. Soft wax is produced in varying quantities in different people and if it accumulates it becomes dry, hard and immobile and may cause irritation or impair hearing.

HOME TREATMENT

- Do not put cotton wool buds, hair grips, or paper clips into the ear to remove wax – since the delicate ear drum may be damaged or perforated.
- Wax can be removed by adding a few drops of warm olive oil to the ear canal two times a day, morning and night for a few days. A cotton wool plug will help to keep the oil in the ear canal.
- Several proprietary wax softening drops are available – ask your pharmacist for his advice.

SEEK MEDICAL ADVICE

- If symptoms persist beyond a week.
- Your doctor or nurse may syringe the ear canal with warm water to remove the wax. The wax is often softened first with ear drops.

EARACHE

DEFINITION

- Earache is a very common symptom in children and can be caused by many conditions, such as pain outside the ear as in the jaw or teeth, or by infection in the ear itself.

HOME TREATMENT

- Inflammation of the ear canal – do not scratch the ear canal and avoid letting the inside of the ear stay wet or soapy after swimming or washing.
- Apply a warm hot water bottle or pad to the affected ear.
- Do not use ear drops without seeking the advice of your pharmacist or doctor.
- Take painkillers for example paracetamol or aspirin until the symptoms subside.
- Do not push cotton buds into the ear canal.

SEEK MEDICAL ADVICE

- If symptoms persist beyond a few days – as an antibiotic may be required to treat an infection.
- If there is a discharge from the affected ear.
- If there is any change in hearing after the earache has gone.

ECZEMA

DEFINITION

- Eczema or dermatitis is a common skin condition in which the most prominent symptoms are redness, soreness, itching and weeping. It may occur on any part of the body but is often seen on the hands and arms. Eczema shows a tendency to run in families and in children, it may occur along with asthma and/or hay fever. Eczema is not infectious.

HOME TREATMENT

- Avoid medicated soap, chemicals or drying agents.
- Wash with bland soap or an emulsified cream to prevent the skin becoming "too wet". Ask the pharmacist for advice.
- Avoid over–exposure to water – wear rubber gloves with cotton gloves inside to avoid hands sweating.
- Dry your hands thoroughly after washing them and apply a bland hand cream to protect the skin.
- In summer wear light cotton clothing.
- Cut childrens fingernails short to help minimise scratching.
- You may be allergic to something in your diet or an external irritant such as copper or nickel bracelets or suspenders or a new perfume. Washing and soap powders are also common irritants. Try and identify these "trigger factors" and avoid them.
- The vast majority of infantile eczemas improve and clear before adult life.

SEEK MEDICAL ADVICE

- If eczema is widespread or not responding to home treatment.
- Your doctor may give you a cream, ointment or lotion containing a steroid. Follow his instructions carefully and do not apply thickly.

EYE, FOREIGN BODY IN

DEFINITION

- The commonest cause of a foreign body in the eye is dust blown in by the wind. Scale or metal from unprotected welding or grinding stone or brick from building works are other causes.

HOME TREATMENT

- Pull down the lower eyelid and remove the foreign body with the corner of a handkerchief or a wisp of cotton wool. If the particle will not come off the eye seek urgent medical advice
- Do not rub the eye.
- Gently wash the eye out with water or a weak salt solution (one level teaspoonful of salt to a pint of boiled water) or use a proprietary eye lotion.
- After washing the eye get someone to inspect it carefully, in a good light, to make sure no particles are left.
- For caustic material in the eye, wash eye immediately using lots of water.

SEEK MEDICAL ADVICE

- If any caustic material is splashed in the eye – after first aid go straight to the nearest hospital accident– emergency department.
- If any particle hits the eye with great force –go straight to the nearest hospital.
- If washing out the eye does not remove the foreign body; if there is any problem with vision or the eye is bloodshot.

EYE, STICKY (BLEPHARITIS)

DEFINITION

- Blepharitis is infection or inflammation of the eyelids. It is commonly associated with dandruff of the scalp.

HOME TREATMENT

- In babies and children, keep eyelids clean by bathing with cotton wool and warm water or a proprietary eye lotion.
- Vaseline applied to the eyelids is helpful.
- In adults, control dandruff by frequent shampooing with medicated preparation, containing selenium or a tar derivative – ask your pharmacist for his advice.
- Remove all crusts and discharge from the lashes by gentle bathing with warm water, eye lotion, or a tepid solution of salt water (one teaspoonful of salt to one pint of water).

SEEK MEDICAL ADVICE

- If a baby is born with or develops a sticky eye, as the discharge may be a result of a blocked tear duct or infection.
- If the discharge is thick and yellow or green.
- The doctor may prescribe an antibiotic ointment to be massaged into the lid margins.

FAINTING

DEFINITION

- Fainting is caused by a sudden drop in blood pressure which reduces the blood supply to the brain and produces a short period of unconsciousness.
- Slight giddiness, cold sweat or nausea may all precede a faint and give a warning.

HOME TREATMENT

- If prone to faints avoid situations that may bring them on e.g. a hot room, going without breakfast, emotional upsets, sudden changes of posture etc.
- If you get warning feelings of faintness or dizziness, sit down with the head between your legs or lie down.
- If person faints – lie them down flat, loosen clothing round neck and chest, raise the legs a little and wait for recovery.
- Make sure the patient's airway is clear – pull the jaw forwards and upwards.
- Do not try to give drink while in a faint and do not try to force the mouth open.
- Give sips of water when the patient comes round.

SEEK MEDICAL ADVICE

- If faints are frequent, as blood pressure should be checked.
- If fainting is accompanied by any unusual features such as chest pain, convulsions, wetting oneself, headache or persistent weakness afterwards.

FEVER

DEFINITION

- Normal body temperature is around 98.4°F (36.8°C). In a fever body temperature may rise to around 105°F.
- A fever usually indicates infection somewhere in the body.

HOME TREATMENT

- The patient should be in bed in a normal, even, room temperature and wear light clothes.
- Avoid 'mountains' of clothes or bed–clothes.
- Maintain a good input of fluids (with sugar and salt) to replace those lost by extra sweating.
- Take painkillers, e.g. aspirin or paracetamol, every 4 hours to relieve symptoms of headache etc. Painkillers will also help reduce the body temperature.
- For children who are hot, keep cool by lying naked on sheets while being fanned or sponged down with lukewarm (tepid) water.

SEEK MEDICAL ADVICE

- If a child has a fit caused by the fever or if the fever is over 41°C or 106°F or if the fever has persisted for more than 3 days.

FLEAS

DEFINITION
- Fleas are small wingless insects which may live on floors, bedding or on domestic animals.
- Fleas bite the skin and produce irritation sometimes causing a rash.
- Cleanliness is no bar to catching fleas – even the most fastidious families can get skin infestations.

HOME TREATMENT
- Check pets and treat them, if necessary with a flea powder available from the pet shop or a pharmacist.
- Fit a flea collar to your pet.
- Treat furniture, carpets, beds, with a proprietary insecticide powder. If in doubt consult the Environmental Health Officer from the local authority for advice.
- Do not scratch the area since infection of the skin may result.
- Calamine lotion will help the itching.
- Irritation may also be relieved by taking antihistamines available from your pharmacist.

SEEK MEDICAL ADVICE
- If diagnosis is not clear or spots are persisting despite treatment.

GERMAN MEASLES (RUBELLA)

DEFINITION

- German measles is a common, mild, infectious disease of childhood caused by the rubella virus
- It is characterised by a light rash of pink spots that usually appears first on the face and then spreads to the trunk where the spots usually merge with one another.
- German measles is not a serious disease but if it occurs in a pregnant woman during the first twenty weeks of pregnancy it may cause serious abnormalities to the unborn child.

HOME TREATMENT

- The incubation period is 14–21 days and the child is infectious from 1 day before to 2 days after the start of the rash.
- The disease often resembles a 'cold' at the start with runny nose and fever.
- Joint pains may develop in adults and are best treated with painkillers such as aspirin or paracetamol.
- For sore throats gargle with salt water or a proprietary mouth–wash.
- If fever present take extra fluids to replace fluid lost by sweating.
- If at all possible keep child away from any pregnant woman. For instance check with your doctors surgery before taking your child in case a pregnant women has an appointment.
- Vaccination against rubella is offered to all girls at about eleven years of age. This should ensure immunity during the childbearing years.

. . . continued

SEEK MEDICAL ADVICE

- If any woman in the first 4 months of pregnancy has been in contact with a case of German measles.
- Women who have not been immunised against rubella or can't remember whether they have should have a blood test to determine if they are immune to rubella. If they are not immune they should always be immunised at least three months before starting a family.

GLANDULAR FEVER

DEFINITION

- Glandular fever is a virus infection of children and young adults particularly among students. It seems to be spread by close contact.
- It is characterised by malaise, sore throat, fever, swollen lymph nodes in the front and side of the neck.
- The illness may linger for weeks and often months.

HOME TREATMENT

- If feverish take extra fluids to replace fluid loss from sweating.
- Bed–rest may be required during the early stages of the illness.
- For sore throat gargle with salt water or take painkillers e.g. aspirin, paracetamol until symptoms subside.
- Observe the lymph glands in the neck over a week or so to see if they are continuing to enlarge.
- The infection usually lasts for 2–3 weeks and a gradual return to normal activities is recommended.
- Refrain from alcohol until fully recovered.
- Take care not to share cups, toothbrushes etc.

SEEK MEDICAL ADVICE

- If sore throat and general malaise are debilitating and long lasting.
- A special blood test may confirm the diagnosis.
- There is no specific treatment other than that outlined above. The illness must simply run its own course.

GLUE SNIFFING

DEFINITION

- Solvent abuse is not confined to adhesives; it includes vapour of many products in domestic and industrial use such as cleaning fluids and polishes.
- It produces hallucinations, dizziness and sometimes unconsciousness.

HOME TREATMENT

- There is no home treatment as such but if you suspect someone is glue sniffing, watch for any of the following symptoms:
  a. Disorientation – a dazed and drunken appearance.
  b. Hallucinations.
  c. Behaviour disorders, eg occasional violent behaviour, or similar.
  d. Hangover effects similar to those associated with alcohol but shorter–lasting and less severe.
  e. Stained handkerchiefs, tubes of glue, tins of polish, plastic bags containing solvents etc.
  f. Breath or clothes smelling of solvent.

SEEK MEDICAL ADVICE

- If you suspect your child of glue sniffing, as it can cause organic damage to the brain, liver and kidneys (occurs infrequently but unpredictably).

HAY FEVER

DEFINITION

- Hayfever is a very common allergic condition in which there is an abnormal sensitivity to pollen, hay or house–dust or other external irritants.
- Symptoms include a running nose, frequent sneezing, itching and watering eyes, catarrh, wheezing and a dry throat.

HOME TREATMENT

- During the hay fever season (peak May and July) avoid walking through long grass, and avoid prolonged contact with grass pollen.
- When you go outdoors it may help to wear sunglasses.
- Avoid any other external irritants that precipitate attacks of hay fever.
- Keep car windows closed when travelling.
- Take holidays by the seaside where pollen counts are lower.
- Keep bedroom windows closed at all times.
- Take note of the pollen count – published daily during the hayfever season in the press and on TV or radio.
- Use a nasal decongestant but avoid over–using – since it may damage the lining of the nose.
- Take antihistamine preparations at night. Some antihistamines cause drowsiness which may be unacceptable at work or when driving. Ask your pharmacist for advice about dosage.

. . . continued

SEEK MEDICAL ADVICE

- If symptoms are troublesome or if wheezing develops with the hay fever.
- Your doctor may prescribe intranasal sodium cromoglycate or intranasal steroids to prevent nasal symptoms.
- If you are seriously affected your doctor may give a course of 'desensitising' injections of pollen extract.
- You may be referred to an 'allergist' or a specialist doctor – to try and establish the precise cause of the allergy.

HEADACHE

DEFINITION

- A headache is a very common complaint. It is usually caused by tension and muscle spasm in muscles of the neck and back of the head after long periods of concentration or anxiety.
- A cold or flu or fever may also cause a headache.

HOME TREATMENT

- Sometimes tension headaches are relieved by simple measures such as gentle massage or a warm dry cloth applied to the back of the neck.
- Take pain killers such as aspirin or paracetamol until symptoms subside.

SEEK MEDICAL ADVICE

- If the headache is persistent for more than a few days or recurs at regular intervals or is associated with other symptoms such as fever or nausea and vomiting.
- Stronger pain killing drugs may be required.

HEAVY PERIODS

DEFINITION

- Menstruation is different for different women and can vary at different times in a woman's reproductive life.
- Excessively heavy periods lasting for more than 7 days or 'flooding' may have no obvious cause or may be caused by a hormonal disturbance or by anxiety.

HOME TREATMENT

- Take more rest than usual during menstruation.
- Make sure your diet is nourishing and well balanced.
- Consider taking iron preparations to replace lost blood and to try and prevent the possible development of anaemia.
- If periods are painful take aspirin or paracetamol.

SEEK MEDICAL ADVICE

- If the bleeding is excessive, interferes with daily living, is associated with clots or is making you feel exhausted. A blood test may be necessary.
- If heavy periods are persistent and a change from the normal pattern.

HOARSENESS

DEFINITION

- Hoarseness of the voice is usually caused by inflammation or irritation of the vocal cords.
- Hoarseness is difficult to treat – healing usually occurs by itself within a few days.

HOME TREATMENT

- Rest the voice as much as possible – do not shout.
- Take plenty of hot drinks or simple cough linctuses.
- Honey in a cup of hot water can be particularly soothing .
- Suck antiseptic throat lozenges or boiled sweets.
- Try steam inhalations or inhalation of Friar's balsam.
- Do not smoke and avoid smokey atmospheres.

SEEK MEDICAL ADVICE

- If hoarseness persists for more than 2 weeks. You may be referred to an ear, nose and throat (ENT) specialist for further investigations.

IMMUNISATION FOR WORLD-WIDE TRAVELLERS

FIRST VISIT
1. Typhoid vaccine
2. Cholera vaccine
3. Tetanus vaccine
4. Oral poliomyelitis

If the traveller is going to the yellow fever endemic zone, he should visit a designated vaccination centre not less than three weeks after the first visit since many centres refuse to give two viral vaccines within three weeks of each other.

The tetanus vaccine advice is for a person not previously vaccinated against tetanus.

SECOND VISIT
This should be six to eight weeks after the first visit.
1. Typhoid vaccine (second dose)
2. Cholera vaccine (second dose)
3. Tetanus vaccine (second dose)
4. Oral poliomyelitis (second dose)

THIRD VISIT
This should be six to eight months after the second visit.
1. Tetanus vaccine (third dose)
2. Oral poliomyletitis (third dose)
3. Normal immune globulin. This is normally given a day or two before departure in order to confer the maximum period of immunity to infectious hepatitis; this is approximately four months.

. . . continued

YEAR OF IMMUNITY PROVIDED BY IMMUNISATIONS

- Tetanus – 5 years
- Polio – 5 years
- Cholera – 6 months
- Typhoid – 3 years
- Yellow fever – 10 years

Further information

- Leaflet SA35 published by the DHSS – 'Protect Your Health Abroad' available free from DHSS Leaflet Unit, Stanmore, Middlesex HA7 1AY
- 'Vaccination Certificate Requirements for International Travel and Health Advice to Travellers' is published by the World Health Organisation (WHO). The DHSS International Division (Tel: 01 407 5522 Ext. 6711) should be able to provide additional information.

IMMUNISATION SCHEDULE FOR CHILDREN

AGE	VACCINE	NOTES
3–6 months	Triple# (or Diphtheria/ Tetanus) Polio	Interval of 6–8 weeks between 1st and 2nd visits
6–8 months	Triple (or Diphtheria/ Tetanus) Polio	Interval of about 4 months between 2nd and 3rd visit (not less than 4 weeks)
12–14 months	Triple (or Diphtheria/ Tetanus) Polio	
13–16 months	Measles	Interval of at least 3 weeks after 3rd dose of Triple/polio vaccine
5 years	Diphtheria/Tetanus Polio	School entry
11–14 years	Rubella (German Measles)	All girls in this age group
12–13 years	BCG (Tuberculosis)	For skin test (tuberculin) negative children only
15–19 years	Tetanus Polio	School leavers

\# = Diphtheria, Pertussis and Tetanus

Pertussis (Whooping cough) vaccine should be omitted if:
1. The child has had whooping cough
2. There is a history of convulsions or an abnormality of the central nervous system
3. There is a family history of convulsions or other hereditary disease of the central nervous system
4. There was a serious reaction following the first dose of pertussis–containing vaccine

IMPETIGO

DEFINITION

- Impetigo is a bacterial infection of the skin that mostly affects infants and children. It appears as a cluster of small blisters. These break, exposing raw, red skin which gradually becomes covered by a golden crust.
- Impetigo is highly contagious – and is spread by touch.
- It commonly affects the face, hands or knees.

HOME TREATMENT

- Take care with personal hygiene, keep towels and face flannels separate.
- Careful washing with medicated (antiseptic) soap is necessary to wash off the crusts and to stop the impetigo spreading.

SEEK MEDICAL ADVICE

- If the condition does not seem to be responding to home treatment.
- Your doctor may prescribe antibiotic creams, ointment or lotion. Gently wash away the crusts with soap and water before applying antibiotic creams or ointments.
- Severe cases may need to take a course of antibiotics by mouth.

INDIGESTION

DEFINITION

- Indigestion or an upset normal digestion covers a host of symptoms such as acidity, burping, heartburn, nausea and occasionally vomiting.
- It can be caused by many factors such as dietary indiscretions, abuse of alcohol, coffee, tea and tobacco and stress or overwork.
- Sometimes symptoms of indigestion are caused by serious disease such as gastric or duodenal ulcer.

HOME TREATMENT

- Regular light meals eaten slowly is a sensible pattern.
- Rest in a chair if the symptoms become incapacitating.
- Avoid fried food and spicy foods e.g. pickles and curry. Avoid tea, coffee, coca–cola. All these foods and drinks increase acid in the stomach.
- Indigestion may be aggravated by smoking or drinking alcohol, especially spirits.
- It is often helped by antacid mixtures or tablets usually taken after meals. A glass of warm milk is often helpful.
- The pharmacist can advise you about the various proprietary antacid preparations available. For example a standard preparation is magnesium trisilicate mixture.

SEEK MEDICAL ADVICE

- If pain and discomfort are severe and recurrent and are not relieved by the measures outlined above.

IRRITABLE BOWEL SYNDROME

DEFINITION

- Irritable bowel syndrome describes a collection of symptoms caused by irregular muscular contractions of the large bowel or colon.
- Symptoms include abdominal pain, wind and irregular bowel actions – sometimes diarrhoea or constipation.
- It is an uncomfortable but not serious condition.

HOME TREATMENT

- The condition is usually markedly improved by a high–fibre diet.
- Eat plenty of:
    a. Raw vegetables (lettuce, cabbage, greens etc).
    b. Fruit – fresh whenever possible, eat skins and small seeds, too.
    c. Wholewheat cereals.
    d. Extra fibre in the form of unprocessed bran – use it to thicken sauces and add to bread and cakes. You may experience excess wind at first but your digestion will gradually get used to the fibre.
- Eat regular meals.
- Drink plenty of fluids between meals – water or fruit juice.

SEEK MEDICAL ADVICE

- If home treatment is not working.
- If you have severe or persistent pain.
- If there is any change in the usual bowel habit or if there is blood in the motions.

ITCHING

DEFINITION
- Itching is a common symptom of many skin disorders, such as eczema, scabies or ringworm.

HOME TREATMENT
- Too much scratching must be avoided as it will only make the itch worse and infected sores may develop.
- Avoid undue heat which generally tends to make itching worse.
- Apply soothing creams or ointments for example calamine lotion or zinc oxide cream.
- Your pharmacist can recommend an antihistamine to help relieve itching.

SEEK MEDICAL ADVICE
- If general itching persists for more than 2 – 3 days.

LICE AND NITS

DEFINITION

- The louse is a tiny parasitic insect that lives in hairy parts on the human body. It lays greyish–white eggs known as nits which become attached and cling to the hairs.
- There are three kinds of lice – body lice, head lice and pubic lice or crab lice.
- Infestation with head lice is very common in school children and the condition is contagious, as lice spread from person to person. Any children and adults can catch lice no matter how particular they are about hygiene!

HOME TREATMENT

- Effective preparations against lice can be obtained from the pharmacist.
- Wash hair with hot soapy water – frequent washing and combing helps.
- After 12–24 hours (depending on which lotion is used), shampoo scalp and comb hair with a fine tooth comb while hair is still wet.
- You may need to repeat the treatment – follow carefully the instructions provided on the container.
- Treat all members of the family and close contacts at the same time if possible – even if they have no sign of lice or nits.
- Regular changing of pillow cases and bed–linen is recommended.

SEEK MEDICAL ADVICE

- If lice are in the pubic hair (crabs) or on the body or if home treatment of head lice is not successful.

MEASLES

DEFINITION

- Measles is a common infectious disease caused by a virus. It is characterised by catarrh, sore throat and a fine pink–red rash over the whole body.
- The illness is usually mild and is most common in the school aged child.

HOME TREATMENT

- The incubation period is 7–21 days and measles is infectious from the onset of the fever until 5 days after the rash appears.
- For 1–2 days before the rash tiny white spots (known as Koplik's spots) may be seen inside the lining of the cheek opposite the double teeth
- Treat as for fever, give aspirin or paracetamol, and plenty of cool drinks to help to bring the temperature down.
- Keep infectious child away from children and from adults who have not had measles until the end of the contagious period – usually about one week after the start of the rash.
- There is no drug that will kill the virus and antibiotics are of no use unless there is also a bacterial infection of the middle ear or the lungs.
- Measles is less common nowadays because many children have been routinely immunised in childhood.

SEEK MEDICAL ADVICE

- If headache and vomiting, or earache develop and child is ill.
- If there seems to be difficulty with breathing.
- If cough becomes worse and more productive or is associated with wheezing.

MENOPAUSE

DEFINITION

- Menopause refers to the time when regular periods stop or become irregular, usually between 40–60 years.
- The most common symptoms experienced during the menopause are; hot flushes, depression, sweating, insomnia, fatigue, headaches and a dry vagina.

HOME TREATMENT

- For headache take aspirin or paracetamol.
- Share your worries – enlist the help of the family, especially for symptoms of depression or anxiety.
- If hot flushes are a problem, wear cotton clothes and try to keep cool.
- If the vagina is dry, especially during sexual intercourse, then use a lubricant jelly such as lubricating KY Jelly – ask the pharmacist for advice.
- Women under 50 should continue with contraceptive precautions until 2 period–free years have passed; over 50's until there has been 1 period–free year. This is because egg formation (ovulation) can occur some months after the last period.

SEEK MEDICAL ADVICE

- If you have bleeding between periods, after intercourse or after a gap or more than 6 months. A vaginal examination and, possibly, a smear test may be needed.
- If you suffer from severe and persistent symptoms such as hot flushes or sweats, as the doctor may prescribe some medicines or hormone replacement therapy.
- If you develop severe or persistent depression.
- If your vagina becomes very dry or sore, a cream containing hormones, or a simple lubricating cream may be prescribed.

MIGRAINE

DEFINITION

- Migraine is a common condition where a person suffers recurrent and severe headaches often accompanied by nausea or vomiting and disturbed vision.
- Migraine attacks frequently occur on one side of the head during an attack and are often preceded by visual disorders such as seeing 'stars' or 'flashing lights'.
- Migraine is caused by constriction and then relaxation of blood vessels in the brain.

HOME TREATMENT

- Lie down in a quiet, darkened room.
- Avoid any known trigger factors of migraine for example chocolate, cheese, alcohol and red wine, shellfish etc.
- Try and relax as much as possible – take regular exercise such as swimming or yoga.
- During an attack take effervescent aspirin or paracetamol.
- Seek the advice of your pharmacist on proprietary medicines that reduce the incidence of attacks.
- The oral contraceptive pill may cause migraine – seek your doctor's advice if necessary.

SEEK MEDICAL ADVICE

- If the attacks are not responding to home treatment or if the attacks are very frequent – more than three per month.

MOLES

DEFINITION
- Moles are defects in the skin caused by pigment–producing cells becoming concentrated in one place.
- They are usually brown/black and may be both in the skin and raised above the skin.
- Moles are common – most adults have an average of 10 to 15 moles. They can develop/be on any part of body.
- Very rarely moles undergo a cancerous change.

HOME TREATMENT
- Every few months check moles to look for any changes.
- Always use a sun–screen cream, not an oil as problems with moles can result from the sun's ultravoilet rays.

SEEK MEDICAL ADVICE
- If a mole is irritated by clothes, eg bra-straps. It may need to be surgically removed.
- If it causes considerable embarrassment.
- If a mole undergoes any sudden change in size or colour, if it itches, or bleeds or ulcerates.

MOUTH ULCERS

DEFINITION

- Mouth ulcers or aphthous ulcers may be caused by trauma, but often they appear for no obvious reason and are thought to be caused by viruses.
- The ulcer is usually white and painful.

HOME TREATMENT

- Ensure teeth and gums are healthy and that dentures fit properly.
- Stop smoking.
- Avoid sharp acid foods and curries.
- Apply painkilling ointment, or suck lozenges. Ask your pharmacist for advice.
- Antiseptic mouthwashes or pastilles will reduce the inflammation.
- Mouth ulcers usually heal by themselves.

SEEK MEDICAL ADVICE

- If ulcers have not disappeared within a few weeks or if there are any other serious symptoms.

DEFINITION

- Mumps is a virus infection usually of young children that causes swelling of the salivary glands. It has an incubation period of 12–21 days.
- The child is infectious until swelling of the salivary glands has subsided.
- The mumps virus is not as infectious as measles or chickenpox.

HOME TREATMENT

- Bed–rest may be needed during the early stages of the illness.
- Sucking ice or ice–cream can relieve discomfort.
- If fever present, give extra drinks to replace fluid lost by sweating.
- If painful give painkillers, e.g. aspirin or paracetamol until symptoms subside.
- If there is difficulty with eating, give a liquid diet for a few days.
- As far as possible keep infectious child from adults who have not had mumps, as the most serious complication in adults is inflammation of the testicles of males and of the ovaries in women.

SEEK MEDICAL ADVICE

- If complicated by headache, nausea and vomiting, sore throat or neck, or by confusion or fits.
- If testicles become very painful or swollen.

MUSCLE PAIN

DEFINITION

- Most commonly muscle pains (myalgia) are caused by sprains or by viral infections such as those viruses that cause the common cold or flu.

HOME TREATMENT

- Avoid the activity that caused the strain for a few days but otherwise keep active.
- Remember both rest and exercise are important.
- Warm baths and exercises for gently stretching the affected muscles can be helpful.
- Apply some sort of heat (hot water bottle, hot bath) to the affected area. Commercial thermal packs are also available.
- Embrocations and sprays may provide relief.
- Gently massage the affected area.
- If painful take either aspirin, ibuprofen or paracetamol until the symptoms subside.

SEEK MEDICAL ADVICE

- If pain does not improve after home treatment.

NAPPY RASH

DEFINITION

- Nappy rash is very common in infants and occurs due to chapping and chafing of the baby's buttocks and groin due to the irritation of urine on the skin.
- Occasionally fungal or bacterial infection may complicate nappy rash.

HOME TREATMENT

- Change nappies as frequently as possible usually after every feed.
- At each change wash baby's bottom and nappy area with warm water then dry thoroughly.
- Leave bottom exposed to air often and as long as possible before fitting new nappy with nappy liner.
- Nappies should be washed thoroughly in soap powder not detergent. Soak soiled nappies in an antiseptic solution.
- Use simple barrier creams such as zinc and castor oil, or silicone creams every time baby is changed.
- Application of a non–medicated talcum powder is also useful.

SEEK MEDICAL ADVICE

- If self treatment fails or if rash is severe or spreads outside the nappy area.

NAUSEA AND VOMITING

DEFINITION

- Nausea and vomiting can be caused by numerous factors such as disturbance or infection of the digestive system, disturbance of the organ of balance in the inner ear, migraine, pregnancy, pain or drugs.

HOME TREATMENT

- If known, direct treatment at the cause.
- Lie down in bed and rest if necessary.
- Avoid all solid food. Drink water or soda–water, a small amount regularly say every hour.
- After 24–48 hours try soft drinks, tea or coffee.
- If these fluids are tolerated, then try eating a biscuit or some dry toast.
- Gradually return to your normal diet over the next few days.
- Avoid rich, fatty or fried foods for a few days until you are back to normal.

SEEK MEDICAL ADVICE

- If nausea and vomiting are associated with pain or if it continues unabated for more than a day or so.
- If excessive vomiting occurs in babies or infants since they require immediate replacement of fluid.

DEFINITION

- Bleeding or haemorrhage from the nose is fairly common since the blood vessels within the nose run very close to the surface.
- Bleeding may be caused by cold, catarrh, over–sneezing over energetic nose blowing, injury. It may also be associated with over–use of nasal decongestant sprays or drops, bleeding disorders or raised blood pressure.

HOME TREATMENT

- Most nose–bleeds are easy to deal with using simple first aid.
- Sit up (unless feeling faint) and lean head well forward, so allowing the blood to flow from the front of the nose and not down the back which can cause vomiting.
- Use an even and firm pressure to pinch the soft part of the nostrils between the thumb and forefinger.
- Breathe through the mouth while this pressure is kept up for about 10 minutes.
- After bleeding has stopped do not blow the nose for at least four hours and then only gently.

SEEK MEDICAL ADVICE

- If bleeding cannot be stopped or if nose bleeds are a recurrent problem and not associated with a cold or injury.

OBESITY

DEFINITION

- Obesity results from an imbalance between food intake and energy output. It is usually caused by overeating but may be caused by endocrine disorders.

HOME TREATMENT

- Follow a sensible reducing diet – reduce fat and sugar intake.
- Eat slowly.
- Try to stick to a diet and record everthing you eat and drink each day.
- A slimming or self–help club such as Weight Watchers may help.
- 'Crash' diets and proprietary preparations can be both generally expensive and ineffective.
- Exercise is obviously helpful. Consult your doctor for advice.

SEEK MEDICAL ADVICE

- If weight gain is associated with other symptoms, such as breathlessness, joint pains.
- An appetite – suppressant drug may be prescribed but such drugs are not usually helpful in the long term.

OVERBREATHING

DEFINITION

- Overbreathing or hyperventilation is a marked increase in the rate and depth of respiration.
- The symptoms include a feeling of panic, chest tightening, numbness or pins and needles in the fingers and toes and in some people – eventual blackout.

HOME TREATMENT

- Tension and stress can make you overbreathe, try and relax and ignore your breathing and it will correct itself in time.
- If you find the attacks distressing hold your breath for as long as you can or better still breathe in and out of a paper bag for a few minutes. This helps to restore oxygen/carbon dioxide balance in the blood.

SEEK MEDICAL ADVICE

- If you do not understand what is happening
- Your doctor will explain the cause of overbreathing and reassure you.

PAINFUL PERIODS

DEFINITION
- Painful periods (dysmenorrhoea) most often affect young women and may start a few days before a period and last until the period has finished.
- Other symptoms such as tiredness, nausea and vomiting and headache may also occur.

HOME TREATMENT
- Continue with all normal physical activities including exercise.
- Reduce anxiety and emotional problems if possible.
- Take painkillers containing aspirin four times a day starting the first day, if possible, before the pain begins.
- Do not wait for the pain to return or become severe.
- If you cannot take aspirin try paracetamol until the symptoms subside.
- A hot bath or a hot water bottle applied to the abdomen or lower back can be helpful.
- Painful periods usually disappear after the birth of the first child.

SEEK MEDICAL ADVICE
- If self–treatment does not work and the pain is severe and is interfering with normal life.
- The doctor may prescribe different painkillers.
- The oral contraceptive pill may provide relief from painful periods.

PALPITATION

DEFINITION

- Palpitations are irregular heart beats that are experienced as fluttering sensations in the chest. They are often distressing and worrying to sufferers.
- Usually palpitations are not due to any serious disorder but if frequent they may be linked with heart disease.

HOME TREATMENT

- Lie or sit down and relax – a common cause of palpitation is anxiety and nervous tension.
- Avoid too much tea, coffee, alcohol or cola.
- Take a drink of water or lemonade.

SEEK MEDICAL ADVICE

- If you feel generally unwell, faint or light headed or have any chest pain.
- When an attack lasts for an hour or more or if you suffer from recurrent palpitation attacks.

PHLEBITIS

DEFINITION

- Phlebitis is inflammation of a vein occurring most commonly in the legs. The skin around the inflamed vein is usually very tender and red.

HOME TREATMENT

- Apply firm crepe or support tights to the inflamed vein – firm enough to provide sufficient support but not too tight as to be uncomfortable.
- Walk about and avoid standing still in one place for long periods. Movement maintains the circulation in the affected limb.
- A hot compress applied to the inflamed area may help temporarily.
- Take pain relieving drugs for example aspirin or paracetamol until symptoms subside.
- When possible sit or lie with legs elevated.

SEEK MEDICAL ADVICE

- To confirm diagnosis if there is marked swelling of the affected arm or leg and if the inflammation spreads or does not settle within 2–3 days.
- If the phlebitis has followed within 2–3 weeks of a surgical operation or childbirth.
- If you are taking the oral contraceptive pill.
- The doctor may prescribe a strong anti–inflammatory drug.

DEFINITION

- A phobia is an unreasonable fear or dread such as claustrophobia (travelling in a lift, or fear of crowds) or agorophobia (fear of open spaces).
- It is a form of anxiety in which intense anxiety and fear are triggered by a specific situation.

HOME TREATMENT

- Try and reassure yourself that nothing untoward will happen if the fear–provoking situation is faced.
- The sufferers should be encouraged to participate in life as normally as possible.
- Face the situation in small doses so that you can slowly overcome the phobia.
- Talk about your anxiety with friends.

SEEK MEDICAL ADVICE

- If you become so distressed that your fears are affecting your every day life.
- You may be referred to a specialist for psychotherapy or hypnotherapy.
- Your doctor may prescribe a short course of a tranquilliser or a sedative to help you cope.

POISONING

DEFINITION
- The taking of toxic substance by mouth may be accidental, suicidal or rarely homicidal.
- The symptoms of poisoning can be very diverse but there may be nausea and vomiting along with anxiety, breathing difficulties, confusion or unconsciousness.
- Most cases of poisoning can be prevented.

HOME TREATMENT
- Prevent by keeping all possibly harmful substances well out of the reach of children.
- Aspirin and iron tablets are particularly dangerous to children in overdose.
- Even nasty tasting fluids such as bleach, or turpentine spirits are drunk by toddlers.
- If person is drowsy or unconscious then remove false teeth, vomit from mouth so airway is clear and the patient can breathe easily, before putting patient onto his side while awaiting an ambulance.
- Maintain body heat with blankets.
- If person is conscious make sure they spit any remaining poison out of the mouth. If acid, alkali or petroleum product taken then give milk to drink.

SEEK MEDICAL ADVICE
- It is always advisable to seek medical help especially for a child.
- If patient is drowsy or unconscious.
- Keep bottles or containers from which poison/drugs came from for identification purposes.

PREMENSTRUAL TENSION (PMT)

DEFINITION

- Premenstrual tension is a common condition that usually affects all women at some time during their reproductive life.
- Premenstrual tension may occur during the 10 days preceding a period.
- It is often associated with fluid retention, weight gain, headache, anxiety and or depression.

HOME TREATMENT

- Reduce anxiety at this time since PMT is usually worse if associated with other stressful problems.
- Take up exercises, keep fit or yoga for relaxation.
- Seek support and understanding from family and friends.
- Vitamin B_6 – pyridoxine or mild diuretics (fluid removing drugs) daily may help. Ask the pharmacist for advice. Foods which contain vitamin B_6 include nuts, bananas and avocado pears.
- Painkillers such as aspirin or paracetamol may help headaches, aches and pains.
- In some people a reduction in salt intake or using a salt substitute may help.

SEEK MEDICAL ADVICE

- If the symptoms are severe and persistent and do not respond to home treatment.
- In some women treatment with the oral contraceptive pill or other hormones by mouth or by suppository may help relieve the symptoms.
- Diuretics (fluid removing drugs) may help if they are taken for at least one week before the period is due.

RASHES—ALLERGIC

DEFINITION

- An allergic rash is an inflammation of the skin (dermatitis or eczema) that arises from exposure to irritant substances such as soaps, perfumes, solvents, base metals used in costume jewellery.
- The symptoms may vary from a simple rash to a redness and swelling of the skin that is very uncomfortable.

HOME TREATMENT

- Try to identify what has caused the rash (for example cosmetics, plants, soap powders, metals, drugs, foodstuffs) and avoid it in the future.
- Often no cause is found for the cause of the rash.
- Use rubber gloves unless you are sensitive to rubber or a barrier cream such as zinc and castor oil.
- Try not to scratch the rash as it will only make the inflammation worse.
- A soothing cream may help the rash or try using oily calamine lotion.
- If mild, your pharmacist may advise you to take a medicine containing antihistamine, usually before going to bed.

SEEK MEDICAL ADVICE

- If there is any doubt as to what is causing the rash or if the rash persists for more than a few days.
- If there is any swelling round the throat likely to interfere with breathing.

RINGWORM

DEFINITION
- Ringworm is a highly contagious fungal infection of the skin. No worm is involved but a circular rash (ring) is formed which tends to be scaly.
- Ringworm is usually contracted in communal work places in schools, sports clubs etc. Occasionally animal ringworm can be caught from close contact with dogs, cats, sheep or cattle.
- Warm moist areas are commonly affected for example the groin, armpits and the feet.

HOME TREATMENT
- Check pets and have them seen by a vet.
- Check other members of the household.
- The sufferer should have own towel and face flannel and keep them separate.
- Moisture and sweating tend to make the rash worse.
- Wash the affected area frequently and dry it thoroughly. Apply talcum powder if not applying medicated creams or powder.
- Wash bed–linen and pillow–cases.
- The pharmacist may recommend an antifungal preparation such as Whitfield's ointment that can be applied to the rash after a hot bath.
- Treatment must be continued for at least a week after the rash disappears. Ask the pharmacist for advice on proprietary preparations.

SEEK MEDICAL ADVICE
- If scalp or nails are affected because in addition to home treatment antifungal tablets may need to be taken by mouth.

SCABIES

DEFINITION

- Scabies is a common skin infestation caused by a tiny insect known as a mite which burrows into the skin usually between the fingers of the hand or wrist and lays eggs. It may also affect the armpits, buttocks or genital areas.
- After about one month an itchy red rash occurs in the infected area.
- Transmission of the mite is by close contact with infected people or bed linen.
- It is highly contagious.

HOME TREATMENT

- Treatment is straightforward but re–infection may occur unless everyone in the household is treated at the same time.
- Normal bathing does not dislodge the mite.
- Change bed–linen and clothing regularly.
- Have the diagnosis confirmed by a doctor.
- The whole family and close contacts need to be treated with an antiscabies preparation which is applied for 2 – 3 nights after a bath. Follow the instructions carefully.
- Bed clothes and other clothes should be laundered and ironed after treatment. Clothing that cannot be washed in very hot water or ironed should be stored for at least two weeks or so before use.

SEEK MEDICAL ADVICE

- For diagnosis and the necessary treatment.
- If itching continues after a month, treatment will need to be repeated.

SCARLET FEVER

DEFINITION

- A contagious infection caused by bacteria. The disease is now less common than it used to be.
- Incubation period is 2–5 days and the rash is characterised by bright scarlet spots which follow 2–3 days after a sore throat or tonsillitis, fever and rapid pulse.

HOME TREATMENT

- Give plenty of drinks to replace fluids lost due to sweating caused by fever.
- Control fever with regular tepid sponging.
- For sore throat give painkillers or gargle with soluble aspirin.

SEEK MEDICAL ADVICE

- All suspected scarlet fever cases usually require treatment with an antibiotic to prevent potential complications such as rheumatic fever or kidney disease (nephritis).
- The patient should be isolated and kept in bed.

SHINGLES (HERPES ZOSTER)

DEFINITION
- Shingles is an infection of a skin nerve by the same virus that causes chickenpox. It usually affects older people.
- In chickenpox the infection is generalised, whereas in shingles the infection is localised to an area on the body supplied by one nerve.
- The commonest site is on the trunk but the face or limbs may be affected. Severe pain followed by blisters over the affected area are the main symptoms.
- The inflammation usually lasts for 2–3 weeks then subsides but pain may continue for a considerable time.

HOME TREATMENT
- Wear loose fitting clothes to prevent rubbing over affected area.
- Apply soothing creams or lotions such as calamine lotion to spots and blisters.
- A cool bath or cool compresses help to relieve the pain.
- Take painkillers, soluble aspirin, paracetamol until the symptoms subside.
- Adequate convalescence is usually required.
- Try to keep away from children.

SEEK MEDICAL ADVICE
- Always seek a medical opinion.
- Your doctor may prescribe special anti–herpes solutions or tablets.
- Post–shingles pain may be a problem and can last for several months after the condition has disappeared.

SHOCK

DEFINITION

- Shock describes the collapse of the circulatory system, leading to impaired blood flow to vital organs, including the brain and the kidneys.
- Symptoms include: Sweating, faintness, nausea, panting, rapid pulse, pale, cold, moist skin, drowsiness and possible unconsciousness.

HOME TREATMENT

- Get professional help immediately if someone near you is in shock, and carry out the following:
  a. Place person flat on their back.
  b. Ensure mouth is clear.
  c. Keep the head low and turn to one side.
  d. Raise legs (unless fractured) about 6 to 12in.
  e. Keep the person warm and reassure.
  f. If casualty is thirsty moisten lips with water, but don't give anything to drink.
- If breathing has stopped give mouth–to–mouth resuscitation at once.
- If casualty is bleeding control by putting pressure on wound.
- If head or neck is injured keep body flat.

SEEK MEDICAL ADVICE

- IMMEDIATELY in all cases of suspected shock.

SHOULDER PAIN

DEFINITION

- Pain around the elbow and shoulder is common and may cause discomfort and disability.
- Usually the pain originates from soft tissues around the joint and not from the bones and joints themselves.

HOME TREATMENT

- Local sprays or liniments to rub in may help – ask your pharmacist for advice.
- Adequate rest with occasional exercise of the joint is required.
- Avoid the activity which caused the problem (such as squash or tennis).
- An arm sling should be used to rest the affected arm.
- Local heat to the area may speed healing.
- Take painkillers regularly for example paracetamol, ibuprofen or aspirin until the symptoms subside.

SEEK MEDICAL ADVICE

- If pain is severe or persistent.
- If suffering general aches, pains or stiffness for more than a few days or so.
- Your doctor may refer you to a physiotherapist for further treatment.

SINUSITIS

DEFINITION

- Sinusitis is inflammation of the bone cavities which open into the main passages in the nose.
- Symptoms include pain over the affected area (cheekbones, lower forehead), catarrh, foul nasal discharge and fever.

HOME TREATMENT

- Do not smoke and avoid tobacco smoke, dusts or irritants.
- Take pain relieving tablets for example paracetamol or aspirin until symptoms subside.
- Use steam inhalations or Friars balsam to break up and loosen the mucus, allowing it to drain more easily.
- Decongestant nasal drops shrink the lining of the nose and may allow drainage of the blocked sinuses – use for a short period only. Ask the pharmacist for advice.
- Antihistamine preparations may be required to dry up nasal secretions – ask the pharmacist.

SEEK MEDICAL ADVICE

- If you suspect an infection as antibiotics may be needed, or if there is chronic nasal blockage or discharge.
- An operation may be needed to remove a nasal polyp or to clear the chronically infected sinus.

SLEEPING DIFFICULTIES (INSOMNIA)

DEFINITION

- Insomnia or difficulty in sleeping is a common problem particularly in the elderly and the anxious.
- There are two main types of insomnia; delay in going to sleep or waking too early.

HOME TREATMENT

- Make sure your sleeping difficulties are not being caused by an uncomfortable bed or a bedroom that is not sufficiently dark and quiet.
- If you cannot sleep it is much better not to lie in bed tossing and turning but to get up and do something such as reading.
- Sound sleep depends on a regular pre–bedtime routine – taking the dog for a walk, taking a hot bath, reading or even listening to the radio may help.
- A 'nightcap' of a hot, milky drink or a little alcohol may help though coffee, tea, cocoa should be avoided as they may actually keep you awake. Avoid late night eating.
- For occasional aches and pains at bedtime take a painkiller such as paracetamol or aspirin.
- Try to go to bed and get up at about the same time each day.
- Take regular exercise particularly in the afternoon or early evening.
- Try to take your mind off the stresses of the day with a relaxing hobby or other activity.
- Lull yourself to sleep with soft music from a radio, with a time switch to turn if off after about 30 minutes.

. . . *continued*

SEEK MEDICAL ADVICE

- If you have any troublesome symptoms such as cough or toothache that may be interfering with your sleep.
- If you are taking any drugs regularly, since some drugs may interfere with sleep.
- Your doctor may prescribe a short course of a hypnotic drug that may help you sleep better.

SPRAINS OF THE ANKLE OR KNEE

DEFINITION
- Sprains of the ankle or knee are common and are usually caused when a strong blow is applied to the joint. The blow can stretch and sometimes tear the ligaments surrounding the joints.

HOME TREATMENT
- GENERAL ADVICE:
  - I – Immobilisation
  - C – Compression
  - E – Elevation
- Apply cold compresses or polythene bags containing ice cubes (ice packs) as soon as possible simply to help decrease the swelling and pain.
- Apply a crepe bandage or an elasticated knee or ankle support bandage.
- Elevate affected leg and if possible rest it until swelling settles.
- If pain is severe take a painkiller for example aspirin, ibuprofen or paracetamol until symptoms subside.
- Avoid for 1–2 weeks activities which bring on more than mild pain but it is essential to keep the joint mobile by taking regular exercise.

SEEK MEDICAL ADVICE
- If pain and swelling are not settling within 48 hours or bruising appears.
- If it is too painful to put any weight on the leg.

SQUINT

DEFINITION

- A squint (strabismus) is produced when the eye muscles are out of balance so that one eye points inwards or outwards.
- If the squint persists, the development of normal vision may be impaired.

SEEK MEDICAL ADVICE

- Any suspicion of a squint in a child should be referred to a doctor.
- If the squint is confirmed the patient will be sent to an eye specialist (ophthalmologist).
- The child may have to wear special spectacles and/or an eye patch in order that the squinting eye may do more work.
- In older children an operation to correct the squint may be needed – this involves surgery to lengthen or shorten one or more of the eye muscles.

STYES

DEFINITION

- A stye is an infection or small boil at the root of one of the eyelashes on the edges of the eyelid.

HOME TREATMENT

- Do nothing until the stye has come to a head and is pointed.
- Do not squeeze or rub the affected eye.
- Use frequent hot bathings, with a hot flannel, to relieve the pain and help the stye to come to a head.
- Alternatively, swelling and discomfort may be reduced by hot–spoon bathing – wrap a wooden spoon in a gauze cloth soaked in very hot water and hold a few inches from the eye for about three minutes.
- A single stye may be treated by pulling out the affected eye lash with eye tweezers. Get some hep to do this.
- If pain is severe take a painkiller such as aspirin or paracetamol until the symptoms subside.

SEEK MEDICAL ADVICE

- If repeated styes develop.

SUNBURN

DEFINITION
- Sunburn usually produces a first degree or superficial burn of the skin. Fair skinned people usually burn more easily than people with darker skin.

HOME TREATMENT
- Avoid further exposure to sunlight.
- Cool baths or cool compresses may be helpful.
- Use soothing creams or lotions such as calamine lotion.
- Moisturising creams may help prevent peeling.
- Wear loose fitting clothes to prevent rubbing the affected area.
- Take painkillers for example aspirin or paracetamol – the pain of sunburn is usually worse from 16–48 hours after exposure.
- Fair–skinned and susceptible people should use a sunscreen preparation each morning.
- Take special care if holidaying in Southern Europe or Mediterranean areas, since strong breezes can give false impressions of the sun's strength.
- The pharmacist can advise on how much protection each sunscreen gives – the fairer the skin the more protection you need. The amount of protection can vary depending on the brand you use.
- Limit exposure to the sun to 30 minutes the first day and increase by 30 minutes for each day thereafter.
- Keep infants and small children covered and out of the sun since young skin is very sensitive to the sun. Give them hats and apply a suitable sun preparation.

SEEK MEDICAL ADVICE
- If severely burned and uncomfortable and home treatment has not worked.

SWEATING

DEFINITION

- Excessive sweating is a fairly common condition that can be provoked in some people by minor exercise, hot weather or emotional problems.
- Occasionally it may be a symptom of illness for example an overactive thyroid gland.

HOME TREATMENT

- Heat–induced sweating is normal and requires no treatment, except drinking extra fluids to replace lost fluid.
- Freqent washing eg twice daily changes of clothing and antiperspirants are usually all that is needed.
- Under the arms – wear sleeveless tops and avoid overuse of underarm deodorants.
- Avoid rubber soled shoes and go barefoot or wear sandals whenever possible.
- Prickly heat – wear little and loose clothing and use fans to cool the skin surface.
- Your pharmacist will advise you on other proprietary preparations that are available to prevent excessive sweating.

SEEK MEDICAL ADVICE

- If sweating is not helped by simple measures.
- In extreme cases an operation (called sympathectomy) can be performed.

TENNIS ELBOW

DEFINITION

- Tennis elbow is a strain of the muscles which cock the wrist backwards. It can affect anyone but is most often experienced by athletes following excessive use of the forearm.
- A small tear occurs in the tendon where the lower arm muscle is attached to the outer part of the elbow.
- The resulting inflammation produces severe pain on the outer side of the arm especially with movements requiring the hand to be turned on its palm, e.g. pouring from a teapot.

HOME TREATMENT

- Symptoms do tend to come and go and will generally clear up permanently after about two months or so.
- When painful, rest the affected joint and avoid arm movements that make the pain worse.
- Tennis elbow splints are available at pharmacies.
- Take pain–relieving drugs for example aspirin, ibuprofen or paracetamol until the symptoms subside.
- Heat and manipulation may be helpful.

SEEK MEDICAL ADVICE

- If there is severe or persistent pain.
- An injection of a local anaesthetic/steroid drug into the most tender spot may be required. The pain may be worse for up to 24 hours after the injection before any improvement is seen.

SORE–THROAT

DEFINITION
- A sore throat is an extremely common condition especially preceding a cold or flu.
- Only about 20% of sore throats are caused by bacteria and an antibiotic may not always be needed. Viruses cause about 80% of all sore throats.

HOME TREATMENT
- Many cases of sore throat heal themselves within a few days.
- Take plenty of soothing drinks and/or ice–cream.
- Take painkillers for example paracetamol or aspirin until symptoms subside.
- Suck antiseptic throat lozenges or pastilles – ask your pharmacist for advice.
- Rest only if feverish or feeling ill.
- Relieve the inflammation by gargling with an antiseptic mouth wash or gargle with soluble aspirin, swallowing the mixture after gargling.

SEEK MEDICAL ADVICE
- If you have white pus–like patches on your tonsils.
- If condition is getting worse instead of better aftcr 3–4 days.
- If recurrent attacks occur or if you are feeling generally unwell.

INGROWING TOENAILS

DEFINITION

- Ingrowing toenails are a common condition and occur when the skin fold at the edge of the nail becomes raised so the nail instead of growing over the skin, grows into the skin, causing pain.
- Can be caused by ill–fitting footwear or by cutting nails down the sides.
- The skin fold may become infected and discharge pus.

HOME TREATMENT

- Good foot hygiene – carefully wash and dry feet and try to change socks at least twice daily.
- Wear good fitting shoes – not too tight.
- Go barefoot or in sandals whenever possible.
- Cut toenails square – if necessary seek the help of a chiropodist.
- Make a V–shaped cut in the middle of the nail at the top edge to relieve pressure on the sides of the nail.
- Infection should be treated by applying strips of gauzes soaked in antiseptic liquid to the side of the toenail.

SEEK MEDICAL ADVICE

- If very painful as an antibiotic may be required.
- Removal of part of the nail or the whole nail may be needed to effect a cure.

TRAVEL SICKNESS

DEFINITION

- Travel or motion sickness if produced when the balance mechanism in the inner ear is over stimulated due to constant motion. This results in too many nerve impulses going to the brain from the ear and causes sickness.

HOME TREATMENT

- Half an hour before you travel take an anti– motion sickness drug or an antihistamine drug. Ask the pharmacist for advice.
- These drugs should be avoided in patients with glaucoma, they should not be taken by a driver or pilot unless prescribed by a doctor.
- Have a light meal only before travelling – definitely no alcohol.
- Make sure children or other sufferers are sitting high enough to see outside the moving car. When on a boat look at the horizon or some visible land.
- Make regular stops, say every hour or so, to get some fresh air.
- Reduce head movements to a minimum – do not read when travelling.

SEEK MEDICAL ADVICE

- If anxiety or emotional factors seem to be the cause of motion sickness.

VAGINAL DISCHARGE

DEFINITION

- Discharge from the vagina is common and the amount of natural discharge varies greatly from woman to woman.
- There is normally more vaginal discharge at puberty, during pregnancy and also for a few days before a period.
- Any discharge which is not clear, is offensive or causes itching should be investigated further.
- There are three main types of infection that cause vaginal discharge: thrush, trichomonas and bacteria.

HOME TREATMENT

- Add a tablespoonful of salt or vinegar to the bath water. Sit in it for 20 minutes. Repeat twice a day for a few days.
- Avoid scented soap, bath salts, deodorants and creams containing local anaesthetic agents because these may cause soreness or allergy.
- Wear cotton pants and avoid nylon pants and tights.
- Avoid sexual intercourse if you feel sore.
- Make sure a tampon has not been forgotten.

SEEK MEDICAL ADVICE

- If the discharge does not clear up in a few days – seek medical advice straight away.
- If the discharge has occurred after you have had sexual contact with someone other than your usual partner – you may be referred to a special hospital clinic for treatment.
- If the discharge is not normal or if it becomes offensive and unpleasant, bloodstained, itchy and sore.
- The doctor can prescribe vaginal pessaries, cream or other suitable preparations.

VARICOSE VEINS

DEFINITION

- Varicose veins are distorted swollen surface veins found usually in the legs.
- They may be caused as a result of pregnancy or to a weakness in the valves in the veins.
- Symptoms include aching legs, swollen ankles, eczema and sometimes ulceration of the area of skin covering the varicose veins.

HOME TREATMENT

- Varicose veins of pregnancy – usually return to normal after birth of the child.
- Wear elastic tights to support the veins – these must be worn all day, well above the site of the highest varicose vein.
- Avoid standing for long periods – raise legs above chest level whenever possible as this ensures good drainage from the ankles and feet.
- Walking for longish periods is useful since this encourages blood flow in the leg muscles.
- Avoid constipation and try and lose weight if you are overweight.

SEEK MEDICAL ADVICE

- If varicose veins are uncomfortable and not responding to home treatment.
- Your doctor may refer you to a specialist who may inject the affected veins to make them collapse. Alternatively you may require an operation to remove the vein/s.
- If ulcers or eczema develop around the veins.

WARTS AND VERRUCAS

DEFINITION

- Warts are caused by a virus and can occur on any part of the body – a wart on the sole of the foot is called a verruca. Warts are slightly contagious and may be spread by touch or contact.
- Warts usually clear up by themselves especially in children.

HOME TREATMENT

- Many treatments have poorer results than no treatment or simple suggestion therapy such as 'selling' the warts to someone for say 10p each wart.
- Treatment may be painful though the warts are themselves usually painless.
- Warts may return after treatment.
- Do not scratch warts since this may encourage spread.
  COMMON WARTS
- Paint wart with a proprietary solution – ask your pharmacist. Do not apply the pastes and paints to normal skin. Continue treatment for 2–3 weeks.
  VERRUCAS
- Cover with non porous plaster when swimming, and emery board/nail file removal of dry skin around warts. Apply pastes or paint to the verruca – ask your pharmacist for advice.
- Do not go barefoot in public places such as swimming pools and gymnasiums.

SEEK MEDICAL ADVICE

- If warts are on the face or genital region or if a painful verruca does not respond to home–treatment.
- Warts can be removed by freezing with either dry ice or liquid nitrogen or they may need to be removed surgically.

WEAKNESS AND FATIGUE

DEFINITION

- Tiredness and lack of energy are common complaints. The majority of cases usually have no physical cause except perhaps after a viral infection such as the common cold or flu.

HOME TREATMENT

- Reflect on the possible cause of fatigue – could it be related to boredom, or unhappiness or a 'stress' at home or at work.
- Eat a balanced diet – extra vitamins and minerals in the form of tonics are probably of little value.
- Pep–pills and tranquilisers are generally of little value and are not advised.
- Take plenty of fresh air and exercise such as long walks.

SEEK MEDICAL ADVICE

- If listlessness continues without obvious cause.
- Your doctor may arrange a blood test to check for anaemia and thyroid function.
- If you are anaemic your doctor may decide to prescribe a course of an iron preparation.

WHEEZING

DEFINITION

- Wheezing can be caused by asthma and may be associated with a cough caused by a chest infection.
- A doctor should always be consulted straight away.
- It is always abnormal.

HOME TREATMENT

- Rest in a comfortable position, sitting slightly forward is usually best.
- Try to relax and keep as calm as you can.
- Stop smoking.
- Take plenty of drinks – water or fruit juices.
- If asthma or hay–fever sufferer then take your usual medication.

SEEK MEDICAL ADVICE

- Always seek medical advice if the onset of the attack is sudden and severe or if the attacks are recurrent, even though mild and short lasting.

WHOOPING COUGH (PERTUSSIS)

DEFINITION

- Whooping cough is a highly infectious bacterial illness particularly dangerous to children.
- The disease usually occurs in epidemics and the incubation period is about 2 weeks.
- Early symptoms are that of a flu but later a cough may develop and the breath is drawn in as a 'whoop'.
- By the time the child 'whoops' he/she is not infectious.

HOME TREATMENT

- A warm, humid atmosphere (steam in the bathroom or kitchen) will help relieve coughing spasms.
- Sleep at night may be helped by an antihistamine–containing cough medicine – ask the pharmacist for advice.
- If vomiting is troublesome at the end of coughing, meals should be kept small and given frequently.
- Keep the child away from cigarette smoke.

SEEK MEDICAL ADVICE

- Always seek a medical opinion.
- Vaccination is highly effective and much less risky than the disease itself, which may require intensive care in a hospital and long term follow–up.
- Epidemics of whooping cough cause considerably more damage than the vaccine. You can discuss this with your doctor.

WORMS (THREADWORMS)

DEFINITION

- Threadworms or pinworms are about 1/4 inch long and look like small threads of white cotton. They are quite common in the stools of children especially school–children.
- The worms live in the lower bowel and emerge at night through the anus to lay eggs which may cause severe itching.

HOME TREATMENT

- Avoid scratching around the anal area, keep fingernails short and wear underpants or pyjama bottoms in bed.
- Good hygiene – wash hands after going to the toilet and before eating or preparing food.
- Bathe daily to remove eggs deposited around the anal area.
- Your pharmacist can provide medication that will need to be taken by the whole family to eradicate the infection. Treatment may need to be repeated two weeks later.

SEEK MEDICAL ADVICE

- If home–treatment fails and worms recur.

APPENDICES

MEDICINE KIT

Keep your Medicine Kit with the items needed for common complaints or for an emergency. The basic minimum list for all homes includes:

For Adults
- Paracetamol or aspirin tablets
- An antacid for example magnesium trisilicate
- A diarrhoea preparation for example kaolin and morphine
- A cleansing agent for example hydrogen peroxide solution
- An antiseptic cream
- Calamine lotion

For Children and Babies, also keep:
- Paediatric paracetamol elixir,
- Zinc and castor oil cream

The First–Aid Kit
You can make up your own First–Aid box or you can buy the complete kit from most chemists. The contents should include:
- Adhesive waterproof plasters – assorted sizes
- Small, medium and large sterilised wound dressings
- One spool of adhesive plaster
- One packet of absorbant, sterilised cotton wool
- Sterilised eye pad
- Safety pins
- Triangular bandage
- Roll of crepe bandage
- Small scissors
- Pen torch

NORMAL HEIGHTS AND WEIGHTS OF CHILDREN

Age in Years	Boys				Girls			
	Height		Weight		Height		Weight	
	in.	cm.	lb.	kg.	in.	cm.	lb.	kg.
1	29.6	75.2	22.2	10.1	29.2	74.2	21.5	9.8
2	34.4	87.5	27.7	12.6	34.1	86.6	27.1	12.3
3	37.9	96.2	32.2	14.6	37.7	95.7	31.8	14.4
4	40.7	103.4	36.4	16.5	40.6	103.2	36.2	16.4
5	43.8	111.3	42.8	19.4	43.2	109.7	41.4	18.8
6	46.3	117.5	48.3	21.9	45.6	115.9	46.5	21.1
7	48.9	124.1	54.1	24.5	48.1	122.3	52.2	23.7
8	51.2	130.0	60.1	27.3	50.4	128.0	58.1	26.3
9	53.3	135.5	66.0	29.9	52.3	132.9	63.8	28.9
10	55.2	140.3	71.9	32.6	54.6	138.6	70.3	31.9
11	56.8	144.2	77.6	35.2	57.0	144.7	78.8	35.7
12	58.9	149.6	84.4	38.3	59.8	151.9	87.6	39.7
13	61.0	155.0	93.0	42.2	61.9	157.1	99.1	44.9
14	64.1	162.7	107.6	48.8	62.8	159.6	108.4	49.2
15	66.1	167.8	120.1	54.5	63.4	161.1	113.4	51.5
16	67.6	171.6	129.7	58.8	63.9	162.2	117.0	53.1

NORMAL HEIGHTS AND WEIGHTS OF MEN—
AGES 25 AND OVER

Height in inches and centimeters (in shoes)
Weight in pounds and kilograms (in indoor clothing)

Height	Small frame	Medium frame	Large frame
62	112–120	118–129	126–141
157.5	50.8–54.4	53.5–58.5	57.2–64
63	115–123	121–133	129–144
160	52.2–55.8	54.9–60.3	58.5–65.3
64	118–126	124–136	132–148
162.6	53.5–57.2	56.2–61.7	59.9–67.1
65	121–129	127–139	135–152
165.1	54.9–58.5	57.6–63	61.2–68.6
66	124–133	130–143	138–156
167.6	56.2–60.3	59–64.9	62.6–70.8
67	128–137	134–147	142–161
170.2	58.1–62.1	60.8–66.7	64.4–73
68	132–141	138–152	147–166
172.7	59.9–64	62.6–68.9	66.7–75.3
69	136–145	142–156	151–170
175.3	61.7–65.8	64.4–70.8	68.5–77.1
70	140–150	146–160	155–174
177.8	63.5–68	66.2–72.6	70.3–78.9
71	144–154	150–165	159–179
180.3	65.3 69.9	68–74.8	72.1–81.2
72	148–158	154–170	164–184
182.9	67.1–71.7	69.9–77.1	74.4–83.5
73	152–162	158–175	168–189
185.4	68.9–73.5	71.7–79.4	76.2–85.7
74	156–167	162–180	173–194
188	70.8–75.7	73.5–81.6	78.5–88
75	160–171	167–185	178–199
190.5	72.6–77.6	75.7–83.5	80.7–90.3
76	164–175	172–190	182–204
193	74.4–79.4	78.1–86.2	82.7–92.5

NORMAL HEIGHTS AND WEIGHTS OF WOMEN—
AGES 25 AND OVER

Height in inches and centimeters (in shoes)
Weight in pounds and kilograms (in indoor clothing)

Height	Small frame	Medium frame	Large frame
58	92–98	96–107	104–119
147.3	41.7–44.5	43.5–48.5	47.2–54
59	94–101	98–110	106–122
149.9	42.6–45.8	44.5–49.9	48.1–55.3
60	96–104	101–113	109–125
152.4	43.5–47.2	45.8–51.3	49.4–56.7
61	99–107	104–116	112–128
154.9	448.–48.5	47.2–52.6	50.8–58.1
62	102–110	107–119	115–131
157.5	46.3–49.9	48.5–54	52.2–59.4
63	105–113	110–122	118–134
160	47.6–51.3	49.9–55.3	53.5–60.8
64	108–116	113–126	121–128
162.6	49–52.6	51.3–57.2	54.9–62.6
65	111–119	116–130	125–142
165.1	50.3–54	52.6–59	56.7–64.4
66	114–123	120–135	129–146
167.6	51.7–55.8	54.4–61.2	58.5–66.2
67	118–127	124–139	133–150
170.2	53.5–57.6	56.2–63	60.3–68
68	122–131	128–143	137–154
172.7	55.3–59.4	58.1–64.9	62.1–69.9
69	126–135	132–147	141–158
175.3	57.2–61.2	59.9–66.7	64–71.7
70	130–140	136–151	145–163
177.8	59–63.5	61.7–68.5	65.8–73.9
71	134–144	140–155	149–168
180.3	60.8–65.3	63.5–70.3	67.6–76.2
72	138–148	144–159	153–173
182.9	62.6–67.1	65.3–72.1	69.4–78.5

CLASSIFICATION OF DRUGS

Drug	Used to
Anaesthetics	produce insensibility to pain
Analgesics	relieve pain
Antacids	neutralise the acidity of the stomach
Anthelmintics	destroy worms in the alimentary tract
Antiamoebics	treat amoebic dysentry
Antibiotics	inhibit growth of bacteria
Anticoagulants	increase blood clotting time
Anticonvulsants	decrease motor activity of nervous system
Antidepressants	treat depression
Antihistamines	treat allergy
Antipyretics	reduce temperature
Antiseptics	prevent multiplication of micro-organisms
Antispasmodics	relieve spasm of involuntary muscle
Antithyroid	inhibit formation of thyroid hormones
Antitoxins	neutralise bacterial toxins
Disinfectants	destroy micro-organisms
Diuretics	increase output of urine
Emetics	produce vomiting
Expectorants	stimulate secretion from the air passages
Fungicides	stop fungal growth
Haematinics	treat anaemia
Hypnotics	induce sleep
Hypotensives	reduce blood pressure
Miotics	contract the pupil of the eye
Mydriatics	dilate the pupil of the eye
Narcotics	relieve pain and induce sleep
Purgatives	stimulate bowel action
Sedatives	reduce activity of nervous system
Stimulants	increase activity of nervous system
Tranquillisers	reduce activity of nervous system

116

SURGICAL OPERATIONS

Appendicectomy	Removal of appendix
Cholecystectomy	Removal of gall bladder
Circumcision	Removal of the foreskin
Colostomy	Making an opening into the colon
Curettage	Scraping the lining of the uterus
Episiotomy	Incision of the vulval area during childbirth
Gastrectomy	Removal of the part of the stomach
Gastroenterostomy	Making an opening between the stomach and small intestine
Gastrostomy	Making an opening between the stomach and the abdominal wall
Herniorrhaphy	Repairing of a hernial orifice
Herniotomy	Removal of the hernia sac
Hysterectomy	Removal of the uterus
Ileostomy	Making an opening in the ileum
Laminectomy	Removing part of the vertebra
Mastectomy	Removal of a breast
Menisectomy	Removal of cartilage in the knee joint
Nephrectomy	Removal of a kidney
Orchidectomy	Removal of a testicle
Oophorectomy	Removal of an ovary
Prostatectomy	Removal of the prostate gland
Salpingectomy	Removal of the fallopian tube
Saphenous Ligation	Tying the saphenous vein in the leg
Sympathectomy	Cutting of some of the sympathetic nerves
Tenotomy	Cutting of a tendon
Thoracotomy	Making an opening in the thoracic (chest) wall
Thyroidectomy	Removal of the thyroid gland
Tracheotomy	Making an opening into the trachea (windpipe)
Valvotomy	Incision of a heart valve

SELF–HELP ORGANISATIONS

AAA (ACTION AGAINST
ALLERGY)
43 The Downs
LONDON
SW20 8HG
Tel: 01 947 5082

ACCEPT NATIONAL
SERVICES
(Alcoholism Community Centres
for Education, Prevention,
Treatment
& Research)
ACCEPT Clin
200 Seagrave Road
LONDON
SW16 1RQ
Tel: 01 381 3155/2112

ACTION AGAINST
ALLERGY
43 The Downs
LONDON
SW20 8HG
Tel: 01 947 5082

ACTION FOR RESEARCH
INTO MULTIPLE
SCLEROSIS
11 Dartmouth Street
LONDON
SW1H 9BL
Tel: 01 222 3224

ACTION ON SMOKING &
HEALTH (ASH)
5–11 Mortimer Street
LONDON
W1N 7RH
Tel: 01 637 9843/6

AGE CONCERN ENGLAND
Bernard Sunley House
60 Pitcairn Road
Mitcham
SURREY
CR4 3LL
Tel: 01 640 5431

AID FOR DOWN'S BABIES,
EDINBURGH
13 Lovedale Road
Balerno
MIDLOTHIAN
EH14 7DW
Tel: 031 449 4100

AL–ANON FAMILY GROUPS
UK & EIRE
61 Great Dover Street
LONDON
SE1 4YF
Tel: 01 403 0888 (24 hrs)

ALCOHOLICS ANONYMOUS
(AA)
Gen Service Office
11 Redcliffe Gardens
LONDON
SW10 9BG
Tel: 01 9779

ANOREXIC AID
The Priory Centre
11 Priory Road
High Wycombe
BUCKS
Tel: 0494 23440

ARTHRITIS CARE
6 Grosvenor Cresent
LONDON
SW1X 7ER
Tel: 01 235 0902

ASSOCIATION FOR BRAIN
DAMAGED CHILDREN
Clifton House
3 St. Paul's Road
Foleshill
Coventry
WARWICKS
Tel: 0203 665450

ASSOCIATION FOR ONE
PARENT FAMILIES
(GINGERBREAD)
35 Wellington Street
LONDON
WC2
Tel: 01 240 0953

ASSOCIATION FOR
RESEARCH INTO
RESTRICTED GROWTH
5 Teak Walk
Witham
ESSEX
CM8 25X
Tel: 0376 517030

ASSOCIATION FOR SPINA
BIFIDA AND
HYDROCEPHALUS
22 Upper Woburn Place
LONDON
WC1H OEP
Tel: 01 388 1382/8 lines

ASSOCIATION OF
CONTINENCE ADVISORS
Institute of Urology
172 Shaftesbury Avenue
LONDON
WC2H 8JE
Tel: 01 836 5361

ASSOCIATION OF THE
PARENTS AND FRIENDS OF
SPASTICS
Rotary Centre for Spastics
7 Queen's Cresent
St. George's Cross
GLASGOW
G49 9BW
Tel: 041 332 4616

ASSOCIATION TO COMBAT
HUNTINGTON'S CHOREA
Borough House
34A Station Road
Hinckley
LEICS
LE10 1AP
Tel: 0455 615558

ASTHMA RESEARCH COUN-
CIL
12–14 Pembridge Square
LONDON
W2 4EH
Tel: 01 229 1149 or 01 221 2347

ATLAS NATIONAL ASSO-
CIATION OF BACK PAIN
SUFFERERS
5 Akenside Court
Belsize Cresent
LONDON
NW3 5QT
Tel: 01 435 3309

BACK PAIN ASSOCIATION
31–33 Park Road
Teddington
MIDDLESEX
TW11 0AB
Tel: 01 977 5474

BRITISH ACUPUNCTURE
ASSOCIATION & REGISTER
(BAAR)
34 Alderney Street
LONDON
SW1V 4EU
Tel: 01 834 3353/1012

BRITISH ASSOCIATION OF
MYASTHENICS
38 Selwood Road
Brentwood
ESSEX
Tel: 0277 218082

BRITISH CHIROPRACTIC
ASSOCIATION
5 First Avenue
Chelmsford
ESSEX
CM1 1RX
Tel: 0245 358487

BRITISH DIETETIC ASSO-
CIATION
Daimler House
Paradise Street
BIRMINGHAM
B1 2BJ
Tel: 021 643 5483

BRITISH DYSLEXIA ASSO-
CIATION
Church Lane
Peppard
OXON
RG9 5JN
Tel: 049 17 699

BRITISH EPILEPSY
ASSOCIATION
Crowthorne House
Bigshotte
New Wokingham Road
Wokingham
BERKSHIRE
RG11 3AY
Tel: 0344 773122
Leeds
313 Chapeltown Road
LEEDS
LS7 3JT
Tel: 0532 621076
Belfast
Claremont Street Hospital
BELFAST
BT9 6AQ
Tel: 0232 248414
Birmingham
Guildhall Buildings
Navigation Street
BIRMINGHAM
B2 4BT
Tel: 021 643 7740

BRITISH HEART
FOUNDATION
102 Gloucester Place
LONDON
W1H 4DH
Tel: 01 935 0185

BRITISH MIGRAINE
ASSOCIATION
178a High Road
Byfleet
Weybridge
SURREY
KT14 7ED
Tel: Byfleet 52468

BRITISH POLIO
FELLOWSHIP
Bell Close
West End Road
Ruislip
MIDDLESEX
HA4 6LP
Tel: 089 56 75515

BRITISH SCHOOL OF
OSTEOPATHY
1–4 Suffolk Street
LONDON
SW1Y 4HG
Tel: 01 930 9254

BRITISH UNITED
PROVIDENT ASSOCIATION
(BUPA)
Provident House
Essex Street
LONDON
WC2R 3AX
Tel: 01 353 5212

CANCER AFTERCARE AND
REHABILIATION SOCIETY
Lodge Cottage
Church Lane
Timsbury
BATH
Tel: 0761 70731

CANCER RELIEF
Michael Sobell House
30 Dorset Square
LONDON
NW1 6QL
Tel: 01 402 8125

CHALFONT CENTRE FOR
EPILEPSY
Chalfont St. Peter
Gerrards Close
BUCKINGHAMSHIRE
SL9 0RJ
Tel: 02407 3991

CHARITY COMMISSION
14 Ryder Street
St. James's
LONDON
SW1Y 6AH
Tel: 01 214 6000

CHILD GROWTH
FOUNDATION
2 Mayfield Avenue
Chiswick
LONDON
W4
Tel: 01 995 0257

COELIAC SOCIETY
P.O. Box 181
LONDON
NW2 2QY
Tel: 01 459 2440

COLOSTOMY WELFARE
GROUP
2nd Floor
38/39 Eccleston Square
LONDON
SW1V 1PB
Tel: 01 828 5175

CYSTIC FIBROSIS
RESEARCH TRUST
Alexandra House
5 Blythe Road
Bromley
KENT
BR1 3RS
Tel: 01 464 7211

DIRECTORY FOR
DISABLED PEOPLE
Little Grove
Grove Lane
Orchard–Leigh
Chesham
BUCKS
HP5 3QL
Tel: 0494 782638

DOWN'S CHILDREN'S
ASSOCIATION
4 Oxford Street
LONDON
W1N 9FL
Tel: 01 580 0511/2

EPILEPSY ASSOCIATION OF
SCOTLAND
48 Govan Road
GLASGOW
G51 1JL
Tel: 041 427 4911

FAMILY PLANNING
ASSOCIATION (FPA)
27–35 Mortimer Street
LONDON
W1N 7RJ
Tel: 01 636 7866

FOOD ALLERGY
ASSOCIATION
27 Ferringham Lane
Ferring
WEST SUSSEX
BN12 5NB
Tel: 0903 41178

GAMBLERS ANONYMOUS
17/23 Blantyre Street
Cheyne Walk
LONDON
SW10
Tel: 01 352 3060

HEALTH EDUCATION
COUNCIL
78 Oxford Street
LONDON
WC1A 1AH
Tel: 01 637 1881

HEARING AID COUNCIL
P.O. Box 153
40A Ludgate Hill
LONDON
EC4M 7DE
Tel: 01 638 9226

HEARTLINE
47 Kettering Road
Rothwell
Kettering
NORTHANTS
Tel: 0536 712559

HYPERACTIVE CHILDREN'S
SUPPORT GROUP
59 Meadowside
Angmering
Littlehampton
W. SUSSEX
BN16 4BW

HYSTERECTOMY SUPPORT
GROUP
11 Henryson Road
LONDON
SE4 1HL
Tel: 01 690 5987

ILEOSTOMY ASSOCIATION
OF GREAT BRITAIN AND
IRELAND
Amblehurst House
Chobham
Woking
SURREY
GU24 8PZ
Tel: 09905 8277

INTERNATIONAL
CEREBRAL PALSY SOCIETY
5a Netherhall Gardens
LONDON
NW3 5RN
Tel: 01 794 9761

INTERNATIONAL
GLAUCOMA ASSOCIATION
King's College Hospital
Denmark Hill
LONDON
SE5 9RS
Tel: 01 274 6222 Ext. 2453

LEUKAEMIA RESEARCH
FUND
43 Great Ormond Street
LONDON
WC1N 3JJ
Tel: 01 405 0101

LEUKAEMIA SOCIETY
P.O. Box 82
EXETER
EX2 5DP
Tel: 0392 218514

MARIE CURIE MEMORIAL
FOUNDATION
28 Belgrave Square
LONDON
SW1X 8QG
Tel: 01 235 3325

MASTECTOMY ADVISORY
SERVICE
40 Eglantine Avenue
BELFAST
BT9 6DX
Tel: 0232 663281/2

MASTECTOMY
ASSOCIATION
26 Harrison Street
Kings Cross
LONDON
WC1H 8JG
Tel: 01 837 0908

MEDIC ALERT
FOUNDATION
11/13 Clifton Terrace
LONDON
N4 3JP
Tel: 01 263 8597

MENTAL HEALTH
FOUNDATION
8 Hallam Street
LONDON
W1N 6DH
Tel: 01 580 0145

MOTOR NEURONE DISEASE
ASSOCIATION
38 Hazelwood Road
NORTHAMPTON
NN1 1LN
Tel: 0604 22269/22339

MUSCULAR DYSTROPHY
GROUP OF GB
Nattrass House
35 Macaulat Road
LONDON
SW4 0QP
Tel: 01 720 8055

NARCOLEPSY
ASSOCIATION (UK)
Secretary
c/o Central Manchester
Community Heath Council
St. Ann's Churchyard
MANCHESTER
M2 7LN
Tel: 061 226 2591

NATIONAL ANKYLOSING
SPONDYLITIS SOCIETY
6 Grosvenor Cresent
LONDON
SW1X 7ER
Tel: 01 235 9585

NATIONAL ASSOCIATION
FOR COLITIS AND
CROHN'S DISEASE (NACC)
3 Thorpefield Close
Marshalwick
St. Albans
HERTS
AL4 9TJ

NATIONAL ASSOCIATION
FOR PREMENSTRUAL
SYNDROME
6 Beech Lane
Guildown
Guildford
SURREY
GU2 5ES

NATIONAL AUTISTIC
SOCIETY
276 Willesden Lane
LONDON
NW2 5RB
Tel: 01 451 3844

NATIONAL ECZEMA
SOCIETY
Tavistock House North
Tavistock Square
LONDON
WC1H 9SR
Tel: 01 388 4097

NATIONAL FEDERATION
OF KIDNEY PATIENTS'
ASSOCIATION
Acorn Lodge
Woodsetts
Worksop
NOTTINGHAM
S81 8AT
Tel: 0909 562703

NATIONAL
SCHIZOPHRENIA
FELLOWSHIP
78/79 Victora Road
Surbiton
SURREY
KT6 4NS
Tel: 01 390 3651/2

NATIONAL SOCIETY FOR
PHENYLKETONURIA AND
ALLIED DISORDERS
26 Towngate Grove
Mirfield
W. YORKS
Tel: 0924 492873

NORTHERN IRELAND
POLIO FELLOWSHIP
485 Antrim Road
BELFAST
BT15 6BP
Tel: 0232 779476

ORGANISATION FOR
SICKLE CELL ANAEMIA
RESEARCH
200a High Road
Wood Green
LONDON
N22 4HH
Tel: 01 889 4844

PARKINSON'S DISEASE
SOCIETY
36 Portland Place
LONDON
W1N 3DG
Tel: 01 323 1174

PERTHES ASSOCIATION
49 Great Stone Road
Northfield
BIRMINGHAM
Tel: 021 477 4415

PHOBICS SOCIETY
(AGORAPHOBIC SOC)
4 Cheltenham Road
Chorlton–cum–Hardy
MANCHESTER
M21 1QN
Tel: 061 881 1937

PREGNANCY ADVISORY
SERVICE (PAS)
11–13 Charlotte Street
LONDON
W1P 1HD
Tel: 01 637 8962

PRIVATE PATIENTS PLAN
(PPP)
Eynsham House
Cresent Road
Tunbridge Wells
KENT
TN1 2PL
Tel: 0892 40111

PSORIASIS ASSOCIATION
7 Milton Street
NORTHAMPTON
NN2 7JG
Tel: 0604 711129

RAYNAUD'S ASSOCIATION
TRUST
40 Bladon Cresent
Alsager
CHESHIRE
ST7 2BG
Tel: 09363 5167

SCHIZOPHRENIA
ASSOCIATION OF GREAT
BRITAIN
Bryn Hyfred
The Cresent
Bangor
GWNEDD
LL57 2AG
Tel: 0248 354048

SCOTTISH COUNCIL FOR
SPASTICS
22 Corstophine Road
EDINBURGH
EH12 7PH
Tel: 031 337 9876

SCOTTISH DOWN'S
SYNDROME ASSOCIATION
48 Govan Road
GLASGOW
G51 1JL
Tel: 041 427 4911

SCOTTISH SPINA BIFIDA
ASSOCIATION
190 Queensferry Road
EDINBURGH
EH4 2BW
Tel: 031 332 0743

ORDER FORM

HOME DOCTOR
AN A-Z GUIDE

by Dr. Victor G. Daniels

Organised in an easy-to-read format this clearly written book
provides essential information on the treatment of common
ailments. Each condition is discussed under the following
headings:

- DEFINITION
- HOME TREATMENT
- SEEK MEDICAL ADVICE

HOME DOCTOR Price £3.00 inclusive of postage and
packing. Please complete the tear-off slip to be sure of your
copy.

Published by:

Cambridge Medical Books
Tracey Hall, Cockburn Street
Cambridge CB1 3NB, England
(0223) 212423

--✂---

To:

Cambridge Medical Books
Tracey Hall, Cockburn Street
Cambridge CB1 3NB, England

Please supply . . . . copy/copies of HOME DOCTOR
at £3.00 per copy (add £1.00 outside the UK for postage and
packing).

I enclose a cheque or postal order for £ . . . . made
payable to Cambridge Medical Books.

Name . . . .

Address . . . .

. . . .

. . . .

. . . .